LEGACY

LEGACY

A Black Physician Reckons
with Racism in Medicine

UCHÉ BLACKSTOCK, MD

VIKING

VIKING
An imprint of Penguin Random House LLC
penguinrandomhouse.com

Grateful acknowledgment is made for permission to reprint an excerpt from
"Remarks at a Press Conference in Chicago on March 25, 1966 at the annual meeting
of the Medical Committee on Human Rights" on p. vii. Reprinted by arrangement
with The Heirs to the Estate of Martin Luther King Jr., c/o Writers House as agent
for the proprietor, New York, NY. Copyright © 1966 by Dr. Martin Luther King Jr.
Renewed © 1994 by Coretta Scott King.

Photos from the collection of Uché Blackstock, MD

LIBRARY OF CONGRESS CATALOGING-IN-PUBLICATION DATA
Names: Blackstock, Uché, author.
Title: Legacy : a black physician reckons with racism
in medicine / Uché Blackstock, M.D.
Description: New York : Viking, [2023] | Includes bibliographical references.
Identifiers: LCCN 2023003556 (print) | LCCN 2023003557 (ebook) |
ISBN 9780593491287 (hardcover) | ISBN 9780593491294 (ebook)
Subjects: LCSH: Blackstock, Uché. | Blackstock, Uché—Family. |
African American women physicians—New York (State)—New York—Biography. |
African American physicians—New York (State)—New York—Biography. |
Women physicians—New York (State)—New York—Biography. |
Physicians—New York (State)—New York—Biography. |
Racism in medicine—United States. | Discrimination in medical education—
United States. | Discrimination in medical care—United States.
Classification: LCC R695 .B53 2023 (print) | LCC R695 (ebook) |
DDC 610.92—dc23/eng/20231108
LC record available at https://lccn.loc.gov/2023003556
LC ebook record available at https://lccn.loc.gov/2023003557

Printed in the United States of America
2nd Printing

Book design by Daniel Lagin

To my mother, my first love and the *original* Dr. Blackstock, whose warmth, affection, and love continue to guide me throughout my life

Of all forms of discrimination and inequalities,
injustice in health is the most shocking and inhuman.

—Martin Luther King Jr.

CONTENTS

Introduction   1

PART I
WHERE IT BEGINS

1. The Original Dr. Blackstock   13

2. Something Wrong   31

3. Everything We Lost   49

4. All the Things They Didn't Teach Me   65

5. Misdiagnosed   81

PART II
OPENING MY EYES

6. Homecoming   93

7. Three Patients   113

8. A Tale of Two Emergency Rooms   131

9. Motherhood   149

10. Diversity and Exclusion   169

PART III
UNBOUND

11. Truth to Power 189

12. All the Patients Look Like Us 213

13. Where I'm Supposed to Be 227

14. A Better Way 239

15. The Way Forward:
   Actions Speak Louder Than Words 253

Epilogue 265

Acknowledgments 273

Notes 279

Introduction

When I was a little girl, my twin sister, Oni, and I used to visit our mother at work. Her name was Dr. Dale Gloria Blackstock, and in the 1980s and '90s she was an attending physician at Kings County Hospital Center, one of the public hospitals affiliated with SUNY Downstate Health Sciences University, in Brooklyn, not far from our home in Crown Heights. Our mother worked long hours at her job and so sometimes we'd head to the hospital after school to see her and do our homework. Walking down the disinfectant-scented hallways, our shoes squeaking on the linoleum floors, we'd make our way to the large, echoing cafeteria, where we'd pull out textbooks from our backpacks and settle down to work alongside the physicians, nurses, technicians, and aides taking a break. The staff behind the counter knew us well, especially because we strongly resembled our mother, and would smile warmly and ask, "Visiting your mother today?"

After homework was done, we'd sneak into her clinic to ask for small change to spend on our favorite red Jell-O. She'd hand it to us and, if we were quiet, let us stay and observe for a minute or two as she examined a patient. Our mother was warm, but serious with those in her care. Occasionally, her face would reveal a smile, but more often than not, she was extremely focused on what they were saying and what was going on in their lives. She'd grown up in the same Brooklyn neighborhood where the hospital was located. The daughter of a single mother from New Jersey, raised on public assistance, she'd become the first person in her family to graduate college, and after graduating from Harvard Medical School in 1976, she'd returned home to her community. At Kings County/SUNY Downstate, she wasn't just taking care of patients; she was tending to her neighbors. In her interactions with them, she always seemed to know as much about their children and families as she did about their respective medical problems. When you came in for a visit with Dr. Blackstock, you weren't only having your blood pressure or cholesterol checked, you were also meeting with someone who was going to assess how your whole being was faring. I believe our mother practiced what is now known as structurally competent and culturally responsive care, which means that the entire complex nature of the patient's background and the social context in which they live, work, love, and pray is considered during evaluation. And her patients loved her for it. She was always bringing home little gifts from them—a knitted shawl, homemade cookies or cake, tokens of appreciation.

My sister and I were only nineteen years old in 1997 when we lost our mother to leukemia—and she was just forty-seven. She died too young, but by then her influence had indelibly rubbed off

on us. Our mother's passion for learning, her dogged perseverance, and her commitment to serving her community heavily influenced our own decisions to become physicians. Oni and I both
graduated from Harvard University and then attended Harvard
Medical School, the school's first Black mother-daughter legacy
graduates. Like her, we both went to work with historically underserved populations after graduating, my sister at a hospital in
the Bronx, while I went to train at Kings County/SUNY Downstate in Brooklyn, following in our mother's footsteps. In the years
since then, I have felt her by my side in so many of my own interactions with patients: her ability to listen to and truly care continues to be a model for me. And it's something that our patients are
crying out for, now more than ever.

During the height of the COVID-19 pandemic, in spring 2020,
I found myself working at an urgent care center in Brooklyn, seeing in the region of eighty to ninety COVID patients per twelve-
hour shift. One day, I remember walking into one of what seemed
like an endless number of patient exam rooms to find a young
Black woman in her early twenties waiting for me. She was hunched
over and staring at her restless fingers, but when I said hello, she
glanced up at me and gave me a quick once-over. The electronic
chart said that she was visiting for shortness of breath after being
diagnosed with COVID-19 a few weeks earlier. Although she was
wearing a mask, I could tell from the look in her eyes that she
was scared.

In those pre-vaccine days, I spent the twelve hours of each
shift covered head-to-toe in layers of personal protective equipment (PPE): gloves on my hands, my bulging surgical cap barely

containing my locs, a surgical mask over the N95 covering my nose and mouth, and a clear plastic shield that would often fog up over my eyes. Not only did the heavy PPE make it difficult to move and breathe in the small airless clinic rooms, there was no way for me to express my encouragement to a patient, offer a smile of reassurance or a look of sympathy.

That day, I introduced myself and then asked the young woman to tell me about why she had come in. But before I got the chance to continue, she stopped me.

"Can I ask you something?"

I told her yes, of course, nodding vigorously in case my voice was muffled through the double mask and shield.

"Are you Black?"

I realized she couldn't see my skin color under all the layers of PPE.

"Yes, I'm Black," I replied, hoping she could see the smile in my eyes.

I could sense the tension leaving her body.

"Thank you, doctor," she sighed. "At least I know you'll listen to me."

"I promise."

In that moment, I knew that I was the physician she needed— someone who looked like her and whom she could instinctively trust.

The reality is that patients like the young Black woman in my clinic have much reason to be suspicious of a medical profession that continues to minimize their concerns and, intentionally or not, cause harm. One of the promises in the Hippocratic oath is "do no harm"; however, we know from multiple studies that clinicians have repeatedly caused harm to Black patients by dismissing their concerns and undertreating their pain. The good news is that racial concordance in clinician-patient interactions—the kind that my young patient craved and that my mother experienced with her patients—has been shown to actively improve health outcomes, particularly among Black patients. Studies indicate that Black babies who are cared for by Black neonatologists and pediatricians in their first year of life are more likely to survive than those treated by white neonatologists and pediatricians. What's more, Black physicians are more likely to specialize in primary care and practice in underserved communities where patients are most vulnerable and in need of expert care. Racially concordant care for Black people is a matter of life and death!

The bad news is that there aren't enough of us. Although I was fortunate to grow up with a Black physician mother, it's important to understand that our mother was a rarity, as are my sister and I. The number of Black physicians in this country remains stubbornly low, with only 5.4 percent of all US physicians identifying as Black, 2.6 percent as Black men, and 2.8 percent as Black women—although Black people make up 13 percent of the population. There is actually a smaller percentage of Black male physicians now than there was in 1940, when Black men made up 2.7 percent of Black physicians.

Training more Black physicians is only one of the many solutions needed to address the glaring and persistent health inequities that exist, but we need multiple fixes, and we need them now, because it's not just one thing that is going to solve this. The fact is that since the days, thirty years ago, when my mother was practicing medicine in Brooklyn, health outcomes have gotten worse, not better, for Black Americans. Despite the extraordinary advancements in health-care technology and innovation, structural racism continues to inflict heavy blows on the health of Black Americans.

US data collection on maternal mortality rates began in 1915. At that time, Black birthing people* were almost twice as likely to die from pregnancy-related complications as their white peers. Today, we are in the midst of an undeniable maternal mortality crisis in the United States, largely driven by the deaths of Black birthing people, who are three to four times more likely to die than their white peers. For decades in the US and around the world, maternal mortality rates had decreased due to improved living conditions, maternity services, surgical procedures, and access to antibiotics. However, around 2000, the US maternal mortality rate began to rise again.

Currently, Black men have the shortest life expectancy of any major demographic group. Black babies have the highest infant mortality rate. These horrifying trends were all true even before the pandemic was permitted to devastate our communities, brutally disabling and ending lives and exposing the deep racist fault lines in our society.

What's perhaps most shocking about racial health inequities is that these outcomes often persist across socioeconomic status strata and levels of formal education. Think of Beyoncé or Serena

* Because people of all different gender identities have the capacity to give birth, I have chosen for inclusive purposes to use the term *birthing person* or *birthing people*.

Williams, both powerful, famous, and wealthy Black women who were at the pinnacle of their careers when they had their babies. Beyoncé is a world-class singer and performer. Serena is one of the greatest athletes of all time. Both women are healthy, are incredibly physically fit, and know their bodies well. Both women suffered near-fatal childbirth experiences. Serena reported that her medical team did not listen to her, endangering her survival and that of her child. Beyoncé experienced the same pregnancy complications as other Black women with considerably fewer resources. Even with my two Harvard degrees, I have a pregnancy-related mortality ratio five times that of a white woman who never finished high school. As the saying goes, if you're not furious about this, you're not paying attention.

Since the summer of 2020, there have been increasing general public demands to urgently reform racist policies in this country and a stronger desire and substantial need to start addressing systemic inequities at their root. There are finally discussions within medicine and health care about including education on systemic racism within medical school curricula and the other systemic factors that influence health, like poverty, inequality, inadequate housing, and lack of employment opportunities. There has been a call for health-care institutions to be more thoughtful and transformative in considering how we are educating and training anyone interacting with patients. The health-care system needs to give practitioners of all backgrounds a framework for understanding what Black patients and communities have gone through in this country for centuries and what they are still enduring. There is palpable urgency to move toward a model of structurally competent health care. The framework of structural competency, first described by Dr. Jonathan M. Metzl and Dr. Helena Hansen in 2014, offers a paradigm for training health professionals to recognize and respond to the impact of upstream structural factors, like poverty and systemic racism, on patient health and health care.

But we can't fix the problem until we can see it clearly. It took me many years to fully understand the centuries of history underpinning racism in medicine today. There were many steps in my own education, glaring gaps in my learning and understanding as a young person and student. It took me until well into my career as physician to recognize the sheer scale of the problem, to free myself from the institutional status quo so that I could begin to fully speak my truth. It wasn't until the time of COVID-19 and the Black Lives Matter protests of 2020 that I finally came into my power and truth as a Black physician advocate on these issues. It was also at this time that I began to write this book.

In the chapters to follow, I will trace my mother's journey and my own as a physician, identifying, as I go, the fault lines both within and outside our medical system. My hope is that our story will speak to anyone who is concerned about dismantling racism and centering equity and justice in this country, because it's impossible to truly understand these phenomena until you understand the ways Black people have been excluded, ignored, and ill-served by our health-care system. We can and must do better for our Black patients and other patients of color, and by extension create communities that are fairer, more equitable, and healthier for everyone. Yet, progress has been far too slow.

Recently, I discovered an introductory letter my mother wrote, over three decades ago, for the event program of a 1990 convention of local Black physicians, in which she grapples with so many of the same problems we're confronting today. "It is ironic that as we enter the age of neotechnology," my mother wrote thirty years ago, "we do not have a health-care system in place that is equitable for all participants. Worse, a health-care system that refuses to embrace all in need." Although she died prematurely, my mother's spirit lives on in my sister and me, her patients, the communities she served, the future physicians she mentored, and the organizations she led. It will live on in this book too.

PART I

WHERE IT BEGINS

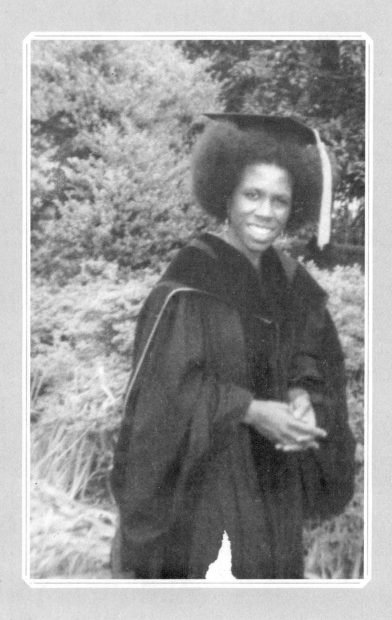

ONE

The Original Dr. Blackstock

From an early age, my twin sister, Oni, and I loved to play with our mother's doctor's bag. It was an old-school, heavy black leather bag, worn and cracked around the edges, that snapped open from the top to reveal the medical instruments inside. Her full name was written in faded golden uppercase letters across one side of the bag, followed by "M.D." The bag lived in her bedroom, under her bureau. As children, we were always getting into her business, whether it was looking through old papers and photographs in the small file cabinet in her room or pulling out shoes and scarves from her closet. We knew that the medical bag was important to her, so that made it important to us.

Whenever we could, we snuck up into her room, emptying out the contents of the bag on the floor: her stethoscope, with its long rubber tubing, the little hammer to test reflexes, the otoscope for ear exams, the ophthalmoscope for looking at the eyes. Then we'd sit and play doctor together. I'd listen to the thump, thump, thump of my sister's heart with the stethoscope in my ears or I'd hop up onto the bed so Oni could hit just under my knee with the reflex hammer, making my leg flip up quickly. If our mother came in and found us mid-game, she would smile warmly. She was a petite woman who wore her hair natural and in a small Afro.

"Girls, please be careful with those. They're all quite delicate," she warned us.

Except for the stethoscope, I didn't know any of the names of the precious contents of the bag, but I understood these were the tools of our mother's trade. By the time my sister and I got to Harvard Medical School, the instruments were as familiar to us as the forks and spoons in our kitchen.

The children's advocate Marian Wright Edelman once famously pointed out, "You can't be what you can't see." Growing up in Brooklyn in the 1980s and '90s, we saw Black women who were physicians all around us. Our mother practiced medicine at Kings County Hospital Center and its state affiliate, SUNY Downstate Health Sciences University, not far from our home in central Brooklyn. Our own pediatrician, Dr. June Mulvaney, was a Black woman. We loved going to see Dr. Mulvaney, even if vaccinations were involved, because she was a bespectacled, kind older woman with soft hands and an even softer smile, who was a good friend of our mother's. Another Black physician, Dr. Mildred Clarke, an obstetrician-gynecologist, lived on our block. We would often see Dr. Clarke while out running errands, stopping to chat about the most recent neighborhood news. Our mother was the president of an organization of local Black women physicians that included Dr. Clarke and Dr. Mulvaney. They were all very put-together, fiercely intelligent women who held themselves with pride and devoted their little spare time educating their community through holding events like local health fairs.

From the day she gave birth to us at Columbia-Presbyterian Hospital in the Washington Heights section of Manhattan, our mother was determined that my sister and I should have every opportunity she had lacked. We grew up in the home our family owned on St. Mark's Avenue in Crown Heights, Brooklyn. Back then, Crown Heights was a bustling neighborhood that was home to many middle-class and working-class families, a uniquely Brooklyn mix of Black Americans and immigrants from the Caribbean like our father, Earl Blackstock, who was born in Jamaica. Our mother was constantly reading to us as small children, bringing us to the library for story time or taking us on educational adventures in Prospect Park and the Brooklyn Botanic Garden. When we got older and entered grade school, she was the kind of mother who didn't hesitate to give us extra assignments if she felt our teachers weren't assigning enough challenging work. If we had friends over for sleepovers, she'd cue up the movie and popcorn, and when the movie was over, she'd announce it was time to do our math worksheets. Our friends, who also had to do the worksheets, didn't seem to mind too much—somehow, she made it all seem like part of the fun. Saturdays were for a host of extracurricular activities: violin lessons, music theory, modern dance, and gymnastics. I can still picture her, leaning against the sink in our old kitchen, scouring the newspaper for educational activities while we were on vacation from school. Her goal was to keep us stimulated—always. Much to our dismay, we were rarely allowed to watch television. On weekends and holidays, we went to the most popular NYC museums, the United Nations, science exhibits, with our mother narrating, explaining, pointing things out as we went along. Even a walk around our neighborhood was an educational adventure, with her perusing her pocket-size book on flowers and pointing out the different types in our neighbors' front yards.

"Girls, come over here. Look at these gorgeous azaleas," she'd say to us, bending down to touch the flowers lightly with her slender fingers. "They bloom only in the springtime," she'd continue as we peered over her shoulders.

Looking back, I think she understood that this world was going to be tough on us and she needed to make sure we were fully prepared, but also that we experienced moments of joy.

For our mother, science was part of that joy. Once we went to a science exhibit where there was a real cow's eyeball on display so that kids could pick it up and see how an eye worked. At first, my sister and I recoiled from touching the large white eye with its spidery blood vessels, but our mother persuaded us to cradle the strange object in our hands, then she leaned in close and explained the mechanisms of the eye to us in great detail. What had scared us a few moments before became a way to introduce us to the wonder of sight.

When summer came around, she signed us up for science programs, including one at her hospital, where she taught some of our sessions. Her specialty was nephrology, the study of the kidneys, and I have a clear memory of sitting in class at age twelve, with a small group of other students, watching her standing in front of the chalkboard, wearing her long white coat over her small frame. I felt so proud to have her up in front of the room teaching a classroom of my peers.

As she took a big piece of white chalk, she asked us, "Did you know that the kidney is one of the most sophisticated organs in our bodies?"

She drew a long looping shape on the board, exclaiming, "And this is the nephron, the smallest unit of the kidney! It's a power-house."

I remember her pulling a cylinder-shaped filter from a dialysis machine, to show us how it processed the blood from patients. She explained to us, in easy-to-understand terms, how this plain-looking filter saved lives. It was in that moment, sitting in that classroom as a twelve-year-old on a hot summer day, that I real-ized the power of my mother's work—to heal, to repair, to care. To be the difference between someone living and dying. I felt in awe of her.

I later learned that our mother chose her specialty, nephrology, because it's one of the most difficult specialties in medicine—the kidneys are incredibly complex organs, and she loved a challenge. But I believe she also went into the field because kidney disease disproportionately affects Black people, and she wanted to help in some way. Because poorly controlled blood pressure and blood sugar negatively impact the kidney's function, many of her pa-tients also had these conditions, which were the result of lack of access to quality care and the chronic pressure of living with racism and other structural inequities. In her work, my mother was determined to address these entrenched health problems to the utmost of her abilities.

It wasn't only patients who benefited from her time and attention. Black medical students and junior faculty at Downstate sought her out for inspiration and advice and she became a mentor to a generation of Brooklyn physicians, even inspiring those in health care who weren't physicians, but physician assistants, nurses, and social workers. Many years later, as an adult, I ran into a former student of my mother's at a medical conference in the city. We made eye contact across the room, and she smiled and made her way toward me, later saying that she had recognized me because I looked so much like my mother. She immediately introduced herself, hugged me tightly, and told me that when she was a third-year medical student doing her clinical clerkship, she had gone to see my mother and confessed how nervous she felt about presenting patient cases. She had explained how she was immobilized with fear and anxiety when it came her turn to describe the patient's medical history and plan for treatment to the team. From then on, my mother met with her every morning, before the start of the day, so they could practice her oral presentations together. This wasn't part of my mother's role or responsibility at Downstate—she wasn't even on the woman's team. But my mother knew how it felt to be a student looking for that kind of support, and so she became the mentor she wished she'd had. Today, that student is the associate dean in the Office of Diversity Education and Research at a New York City medical school.

Our mother was tireless in her work ethic. Even after she left the hospital, her work wasn't done. Back then, she was president of the Susan Smith McKinney Steward Medical Society, a local organization of Black women physicians named after the third Black woman to obtain a medical degree in the US and the first in New York state. During the society's regular meetings, Oni and I would sit in the back of a large conference room, doing our homework, whispering, or passing silly notes back and forth, as my mother and her colleagues handled their serious business. They spent considerable time planning community health fairs, where they would dispense information about diabetes, high blood pressure, and other health issues rampant in our community. At the fairs, they would take people's vital signs, recommend follow-up services, and counsel neighbors about healthy diet and exercise. Our mother and the other women in her organization were our role models. They worked, they raised children, they took care of their households, and they gave back to their communities.

I don't think it ever occurred to Oni and me to do anything else with our lives but to follow in their footsteps.

While Oni and I were surrounded by Black women physicians as young girls, our mother had had the opposite experience. She used to tell us that growing up, she rarely saw a physician, let alone a Black one. Raised by a single mother and without a father in sight, with five siblings, my mother spent her childhood living in what she described as a series of rodent- and roach-infested apartments, including one where a rat had once bitten her on the forehead (she still had the scar to prove it). Back then, the family received support from Aid to Dependent Children, or ADC—otherwise known as welfare—but according to our mother, those funds were never enough. Once, she told us, our grandma was so desperate to put food on the table, she dragged her six kids down to the welfare office and threatened to leave them there unless she could be given more money. Then she walked out. Although Grandma couldn't have been gone for more than fifteen minutes, to our mother, who was six years old at the time, it felt like an eternity.

Our grandmother was a sturdy woman who had a no-nonsense personality and a life story that was full of tough times. For a Black woman born in New Jersey during the Great Depression, the idea that she could have a daughter who might succeed academically and go on to be a physician must have felt beyond her imagination. Grandma had barely completed high school. She got nervous when our mother spent too much time studying and was always reminding her to clean or do dishes, to make herself useful. Yet her influence was felt in the family in other ways. She read the *Daily News* to her children, pointing out words and pictures to them, and it must have helped because my aunt and one of my uncles were placed in gifted programs. Grandma didn't just raise smart children; she was talented in her own right. Years later, she passed the exam to become a licensed practical nurse on her first try without ever cracking a textbook (she claimed she couldn't read the small print). She attended school full-time, worked full-time, took care of her family, and got herself off welfare.

Our mother suffered from a severe stutter as a child. My

grandmother wouldn't have known what a speech pathologist was, and even if she had, she likely couldn't have afforded one. Instead, her home remedy was to slap our mother hard in the mouth with her hand or a comb whenever her daughter stuttered. Eventually, our mother somehow overcame the speech impediment, but in its place, she developed a deep-seated fear of speaking in public, worried that the words wouldn't come out right—or wouldn't come out at all. Even as an adult, a physician and leader in her community, she knew she had to be very well prepared for presentations. She couldn't ad-lib.

She also developed a particular kind of empathy for those who are struggling, a desire to help people, and the drive to use education to transcend her circumstances. At her all-girls Catholic high school in Brooklyn, our mother realized that she probably wouldn't make it as a nun or a saint, and so the next most challenging and interesting thing to do was to become a physician. When she first began to consider becoming a doctor, she went to one of the sisters to ask for advice. She told this woman that she was thinking of trying for a medical degree. The sister laughed at her, despite our mother's excellent grades.

"Maybe you could try to be a social worker," the nun said.

With doubt creeping in, she spent two years at New York City Community College studying liberal arts. It wasn't until she transferred to Brooklyn College, a four-year-college, that she found the support necessary to cultivate her interest in medicine. Dr. Clyde Dillard, a Black chemistry professor, took her under his wing, as he did with all students of color in his classes, eventually becoming her mentor. There at Brooklyn College, she majored in biology and completed her premed courses. She excelled and during her last two college summers, she was accepted to and attended the Harvard Health Career Summer Program, for students from groups historically excluded from medicine who were interested in a future in the health profession. This program allowed her to take courses at Harvard Medical School. Dr. Dillard told her, "I really think you should apply to medical school." Following his sage advice, she did. She was accepted to every medical school to which she applied, ultimately matriculating early-decision at Harvard.

Her first day of medical school was a complete culture shock for her. "What am I doing here?" she remembered asking herself. She was a little Black girl from Brooklyn; meanwhile, the majority of her classmates were white and from affluent backgrounds. In her class alone, there was a student who was a relative of Jackie Onassis, several students whose parents had written the textbooks they were using in class and were professors at Harvard, and another student whose father won the Nobel Prize in Medicine for immunology. Her life couldn't have been more different than theirs. While she wanted to believe that she deserved to be there, she wasn't always certain. Her own claim to fame was that her mother had received her LPN degree after raising six children, attending school full-time, working full-time, taking care of the family, and getting off welfare. Our mother was very proud of her mother's achievements, but they weren't a Nobel Prize in Medicine.

When my mother told the story of her time at Harvard, she insisted that she didn't experience any overt racism while there. Notably, her class at Harvard was one of the most diverse in the school's history because of diversity initiatives begun soon after Martin Luther King Jr.'s assassination. A full 10 percent of her class were Black students. The faculty gave a lot of support to everyone in class, although because my mother was shy due to her stutter, she ended up not being able to take advantage of the help; she was too scared to ask for it. Even so, there were inevitably incidents that led her to question whether racism was at work. During one of her rotations, a professor held open a door for a white male student while letting it slam in her face. Another time, when a male professor made a joke in bad taste about women during a radiology conference, he apologized to a white student within earshot, but not to my mother, who was standing right next to him. Once, during a breakfast meeting, my mother's hand accidentally brushed against one of the pastries and she saw out of the corner of her eye one of the white residents pick it up and drop it in the garbage. Another time, she was told not to sleep in an empty patient room—as was customary after a night shift—because a white male resident needed to sleep there. Then there was the white patient who didn't want to be treated by a Black student-doctor and told my mother this in no uncertain terms. By the time she graduated medical school, she was exhausted.

It had been more than twenty years since Mildred Jefferson became the first Black woman to graduate from HMS in 1951, and my mother was not alone there. Thankfully, she was able to befriend Black classmates at Harvard who supported her, including a young woman named Jessie Sherrod. Jessie hailed from Mississippi and was the first student from the HBCU Tougaloo College, near Jackson, to attend Harvard Medical School. She had grown up picking cotton with a father who was a local civil rights leader and who instilled in Jessie and his other children a very strong sense of self. In eighth grade, her father chose her to integrate a café in her small town of Hollandale, because she was a girl and would be considered less of a threat to the system. Jessie, all of thirteen years old, sat down with a Student Nonviolent Coordinating Committee (SNCC) activist, a white college student, Chuck Carpenter, from Ohio State University, and ordered a hamburger and a Coke and the rest is history. Unlike our mother, Jessie believed firmly that she belonged at Harvard Medical School. These were the kind of friends that carried our mother through the tumultuous transition from the familiarity of home to a place like Harvard, where she felt like a fish out of water.

While I will always want to celebrate my mother's achievements, I feel I would be doing her memory an injustice if I portrayed her story only as one of exceptionalism, of the plucky young Black woman from humble beginnings who through grit and determination rose to success. To truly pay tribute to her, I know I must situate her story within the broader context of the historical barriers that Black people in this country have faced entering the medical field.

For centuries in this country, white-only medical schools, with their exclusionary policies and practices, made it virtually impossible for Black people to receive medical training. It was only after the Civil War, with thousands of injured veterans in desperate need of medical care, that a small handful of Black trainees

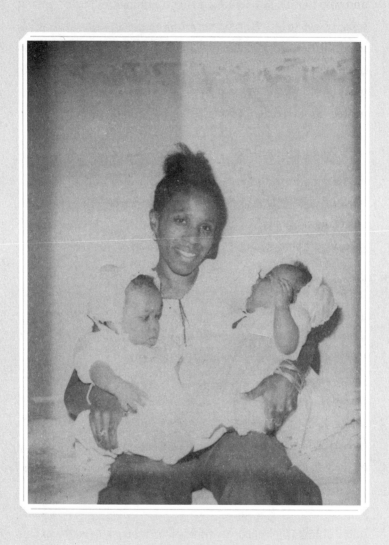

began to be admitted to white medical schools in the North. And it wasn't until Reconstruction that a number of Black medical schools sprang up in the South, enabling us to finally have access to medical training in greater numbers. These schools were Howard University College of Medicine, established in Washington, DC, in 1868; Meharry Medical College, established in Nashville, Tennessee, in 1876; Leonard Medical School, established in 1882 in Raleigh, North Carolina; New Orleans University Medical College, founded in 1887; Knoxville College Medical Department, founded in 1895; Chattanooga National Medical College, founded in 1902; and the University of West Tennessee College of Physicians and Surgeons, founded in 1904. By 1905, those Black medical schools had trained 1,465 doctors. Each of those doctors was poised to train a new generation of doctors, who would have gone on to train a generation of their own.

And then that legacy came to a grinding halt. The reason was the publication of the Flexner Report, a landmark report in US medical history that had a devastating impact on the numbers of Black physicians in this country. Abraham Flexner, the white author of the report, was an education specialist in the early 1900s who was employed by the Carnegie Foundation and the American Medical Association to travel to all 155 medical schools in the US and Canada to assess the state of medical education. His report, which was published in 1910, led to broad standardization of medical schools, with the top medical school in the country at the time—Johns Hopkins in Baltimore—being held up as the example that all other medical schools must follow. The new standards certainly went some way toward elevating the quality of medical care in this country. The problem was that smaller, Black institutions simply didn't have the resources or endowments to implement the more rigorous instruction required by these new standards.

Flexner had strongly racist opinions on the role of Black people in the medical realm. He wrote that Black students should be trained in "hygiene rather than surgery" and were best employed as "sanitarians" who could help protect whites from common diseases like tuberculosis. "Not only does the Negro himself suffer from hookworm and tuberculosis; he communicates them to his white neighbors," Flexner wrote, begrudgingly admitting that Black people did need to have some role in health care, but only as it pertained to whites. "The Negro must be educated not only for his sake, but for ours. He is, as far as the human eye can see, a permanent factor in the nation." He wrote that Black medical schools were "wasting small sums annually and sending out undisciplined men, whose lack of real training is covered up by the imposing MD degree."

After the Flexner Report, five of the seven Black medical schools in America were forced to close down, leaving only Howard and Meharry schools.

Almost a hundred years later, in June 2020, in the midst of a global pandemic and the Black Lives Matter protests, I read an article about the Flexner Report that popped up in my Twitter feed. I wasn't prepared for its contents. My heart dropped as my eyes scanned the information. The article described a new study that estimated that if the majority of Black medical schools had been allowed to remain open after the Flexner Report in 1910, continuing to train Black doctors to this day, they would have educated between 25,000 and 35,000 physicians. In essence, tens of thousands of future Black physicians had disappeared. For context, in 2015, there were estimated to be only 46,133 Black physicians practicing in the US. I remember sobbing as I absorbed the magnitude of those numbers. When my mother died at forty-seven, I remember feeling the loss not only for myself, but for her patients too. They had experienced the care of a physician who listened to them, understood their lives and experiences, and was invested in them as whole human beings. Now I tried to imagine the hundreds of thousands of similar patient-physician relationships that never had a chance to exist at all because of a report that was designed to improve health outcomes, but only for patients who were white. The loss of so many Black physicians to the field of medicine and to our communities has been undeniably profound. We know that racial concordance in patient-physician interactions influences everything from how a patient feels when they leave their appointment to how likely they are to take their medications, and so we also know that had these schools remained open, the health of our communities might be in a different place, likely better than it is today. And because Black physicians are more likely to mentor and sponsor Black students, these students would have felt safer and more comfortable, and would have been more likely to thrive in academic medical environments, resulting in greater academic success and career opportunities.

More than one hundred years after the Flexner Report, we're still recovering from its impact. In 1910, 2.5 percent of all US physicians were Black. By 2008, that number had increased to

6.8 percent. Today, the number of Black physicians in the workforce still remains disproportionately low. In our current times, exclusionary criteria in medical school admissions look very different than they did in the past, but they still have the same detrimental effect on the representation of Black physicians. The modern MCAT, the standardized test required to enter medical school, has been shown to be discriminatory against Black students and other students of color, even as it does a poor job of predicting future success as a physician. Studies have shown that election to the medical school honor society, Alpha Omega Alpha (AOA), which often determines entry into selective medical specialties such as ophthalmology and dermatology, is embedded in racism, resulting in few Black student members. Because academic medical centers receive federal funding for education and training, they have a social contract with the public to ensure that medical schools accept and support a student body that fully represents the communities being served. Some medical schools have recently adopted a holistic review process that places value on lived experience and personal attributes apart from traditional metrics like MCAT scores and grades; however, this process has not been operationalized consistently by schools. Ultimately, this social accountability that medical schools have means investing in the communities that they have a mandate to serve by developing pipeline programs, investing in local, community-based initiatives, and intentionally selecting students from historically excluded communities.

When I was a little girl, and even into my twenties, I thought that our mother was successful because she worked incredibly hard, she loved science, and she was determined. More recently, I've realized that she wasn't exceptional, she was just one of the lucky ones who made it through. The fact is there have always been many "exceptional" Black people like my mother, who never had the same opportunity, who were never able to go to medical school because of systemic racism. For me, my mother's success—and the way she stewarded my sister and me to reach our own success—is a reminder of everyone who's not here with us but who should be. It's a reminder of this tremendous loss.

TWO

Something Wrong

Unlike our mother, Oni and I grew up with a certain amount of privilege. Our family owned our home, so we always had a stable place to live. We were well fed and well clothed—there was always food in the fridge and enough money for winter coats and boots. Even though they were socially and politically conscious, our parents were still extremely focused on our education as a way to achieve success in life. We went to schools in the neighborhood for preschool and elementary, but when we reached middle school age, our mother and father decided they wanted a more academically rigorous environment for us, and so they transferred us into a predominantly white private school about a thirty-minute bus ride away in the affluent neighborhood of Brooklyn Heights, and from there, we went to one of the top public high schools in the city, Stuyvesant High School, across the river in Manhattan.

My childhood can only be described as a happy one, but that

didn't mean there wasn't an edge to it. All around us, there were families in much more precarious situations than ours. In the 1980s and '90s, when we grew up, there was a significant drug element in Crown Heights as crack cocaine flooded into New York City and urban communities across the country. We would often find crack vials in our front yard left there by our neighbor, a very thin, beautiful, dark-skinned woman whose addiction to crack was visible in her skeleton-like frame. Often, we would hear our neighbor and her boyfriend, an elderly Barbadian man, having loud arguments through the wall; sometimes we'd hear things crashing, or the woman yelling outside to be let back in when she'd gotten locked out. At times she seemed agitated, other times almost sedated, but she was always kind to my sister and me, saying hello, giving a smile that felt genuine. My mother never spoke poorly of our neighbor and was never judgmental of her. I think my mother saw clearly that the crack epidemic was a public health issue—even if our government felt otherwise. Thanks to President Ronald Regan's "war on drugs," policing of our neighborhood for drug-related crimes amped up substantially during these years, and mandatory-minimum prison sentences for drug offenses led to an explosion in the nation's prison population. It's estimated that around 80 percent of people who used crack were Black, and so our communities were further destroyed, not just by drug use, but by the decades-long sentences meted out to people who were genuinely addicted and needed help.

As children, Oni and I learned to avoid the main drag to the subway station, Franklin Avenue, because there was so much drug activity there, with dealers on almost every corner. Shootings on the block were not uncommon—I saw two people gunned down before I was eight years old. One time, my sister and I were hanging out at a block party on a hot summer night, playing in the street with other children from the neighborhood, when we heard the *POP, POP* of shots fired. Suddenly everyone started running toward safety. I looked back to see one of the younger men in the family who lived down the block falling to the ground. I remember grabbing Oni and running quickly toward our house. Our little legs couldn't carry us fast enough. The young man died in the hospital later that evening. On another night my father was coming home by subway from a PTA meeting at our high school and there was a shooting right outside the train station—he missed being caught in the crossfire by seconds.

Then, in 1991, when we were freshmen in high school, an uprising broke out in our Crown Heights neighborhood. A little Black boy was accidently hit by a car driven by an Orthodox Jewish person, and there was an outpouring of rage. There were protests, sometimes violent. People were injured. I remember feeling scared and unsettled, like everything was out of control. There had been tension for many years between the Orthodox Jewish and Afro-Caribbean residents in Crown Heights. While in the past my parents had taken us to demonstrations and rallies for social and racial justice, they felt, given the intensity of these current protests, it was just too dangerous to be out in the streets. After that, the name of our neighborhood—Crown Heights—became synonymous with turmoil and violence.

Because of the events happening all around, we were aware of the many ways our formally educated, professional parents kept us insulated from the world, protecting us and keeping us safe. We considered ourselves privileged. It was only when we started attending our predominantly white private school in seventh grade that we learned that there were students who came from backgrounds of much greater privilege than ours. At that time, we were two of only five students of color in our grade and the only kids in our school from our 11216 zip code. I remember looking in the directory of students and seeing that most of my classmates lived close to the school in affluent neighborhoods like Brooklyn Heights and Park Slope. When we went to visit our new friends for birthday parties and sleepovers, we saw they lived in beautiful townhomes, on blocks lined with tall trees with immaculate sidewalks and manicured front yards. These were Brooklyn's "white" neighborhoods, and the residents who lived there clearly did not have the same problems with drug-related crime and over-policing that we experienced in Crown Heights. Our schoolmates were never going to be able to understand what it was like to lie awake in bed hearing the sound of gunshots almost nightly, wondering from where that gunfire was coming and who was getting hurt or killed this time. We never considered sharing these experiences with them.

Despite this, over the course of my childhood, my parents did everything they could to teach us to take pride in being Black. They gave us books on Harriet Tubman, Shirley Chisholm, Malcolm X, and Ida B. Wells. We wrote mini essays about what it meant to be "young, gifted and Black," an expression coined by the playwright Lorraine Hansberry, describing all the ways we intended to fulfill those words in our own lives. Our mother regularly took us to Black cultural and musical events around New York City, to plays by Black playwrights and exhibitions by Black artists. At home, our parents complimented our features and encouraged us to feel comfortable in our skin, and to wear our hair natural, just like our mother, with her close-cropped Afro. When we were ten, eleven, and twelve, during our summers, we traveled to West Africa, East Africa, and Bahia, Brazil (a mostly Afro-Brazilian state) because our parents thought it was important for us to understand and learn about our connections to the rest of the African diaspora. During the height of the Cabbage Patch craze in the 1980s, our mother even stood in line for hours to buy us limited-edition Black Cabbage Patch dolls so we would have versions of the popular toy that actually looked like us.

And yet despite all this, I still learned to feel the sting of judgment because of being Black in this country. My first year in high school, I remember I made friends with a white girl who lived in Park Slope. It was only a fifteen-minute drive from our house, but it felt like another world. One freezing cold afternoon, my friend's mom offered to give me a ride home after school. That day I recall sitting in the back of their car and realizing that I absolutely did not want them to drop me outside my house because I was too embarrassed for my friend and her mother to see where I lived. While our neighborhood was home to many modest homes and yards like ours, proudly cared for by their inhabitants, for every house that was kept up, there would be another one that was tumbling down or boarded up, flanked by an abandoned lot strewn with trash and used tires, not to mention the crack vials in our neighbors' yards. Instead, I asked my white friend's mother to leave me on Eastern Parkway, a main thoroughfare six blocks from our house, making the excuse that it would be easier for them to get home from there.

The fact that I felt this way was so confusing to me. The reality was that I loved our Crown Heights neighborhood, and I loved our neighbors. We looked out for one another; we were a community. If there was alternate-side parking—in which you have to move your car for street cleaning on days the street sweeper came through—and we forgot to switch our car to the correct side of the street, a neighbor would come and ring our doorbell to remind us; when it snowed, our next-door neighbor would shovel our front sidewalk for us. And even so, I chose to walk the six blocks home in the bitter cold, with a thin jacket on. Faced with the stark differences between my white friend's environment and my own, all I felt was self-conscious and ashamed. As I walked those six long blocks, I recall shivering as much from the disappointment I had in myself that I felt this way as I did from the frigid temperatures. When I got home, I never told my sister or my parents, because the shame cut too deep and I didn't want them to feel it too.

Even I, growing up in a proudly Black family, had internalized the messaging that I wasn't good enough, that there was something "wrong" with us. As a child and young person, I knew that the clean and well-kept neighborhoods had white people living in them and neighborhoods with the empty lots and crack vials had people who looked like me. I was absorbing the idea through my pores that if I wanted to avoid crime and drug use, if I wanted to make "healthy choices" in my life, I had to go outside my neighborhood to do so. Every weekday morning, I got up and boarded a bus to go to a school outside the neighborhood. Each weekend we got in our car and went to Park Slope to buy food at the closest supermarket that sold fresh produce. If we wanted to go to a sit-down restaurant, we had to get in our car and drive to downtown Brooklyn, where we'd go to dinner at Junior's Restaurant, one of our mother's favorite restaurants. There was no green space close to our home; instead, we had to walk twenty-five minutes to Prospect Park, the nearest park. Even our closest hospital, where our mother worked, was a twenty-minute drive away. As we transitioned back and forth between our neighborhood and the amenities offered by New York City's "white" and therefore "better" neighborhoods, we were coming to the understanding that a good life was available to us, just not where we lived, nor among people who looked like us.

My father's story has always fascinated me because, unlike my mother, my sister, and me, he didn't grow up in the United States, and as a result, he didn't begin to absorb the impact of this country's anti-Black messaging until he moved here in his late teens, on the cusp of adulthood. Earl Llewellyn Blackstock was born in Jamaica in 1942 and raised in the rural parish of Clarendon, due west of the island's capital, Kingston. The land of his birth was rocky, deemed undesirable by white enslavers, but my father's people were able to plant and grow beans, peas, and cassava. Although they had little cash to buy material things, they raised chicken and goats. More significantly, my father was born in a nation where Black people were the majority, where there may have been Black people of different shades, but he was always among people who looked like him. When he was five years old, his mother left for the US, seeking employment in New York City, and joined her own mother who had migrated to the US in 1923 through Ellis Island via Cuba. His father was a migrant farmworker who would travel to the US to pick apples in the late summer and early fall. My father stayed behind after his mother left, raised by his aunt, a schoolteacher. At school, he was considered privileged because he had shoes sent to him from the US, unlike many of his classmates who went barefoot. When my father was seventeen, the family decided it was time for him to leave the island and come to Brooklyn to be with his mother.

My father arrived in New York City on December 6, 1959, his mother recognizing him from the red sweater she had sent him as a gift. He went to live with her on Jefferson Avenue in the Brooklyn neighborhood of Bedford-Stuyvesant. My father had always been bright. Back in Jamaica, he had kept up-to-date on current events by reading the old newspapers and magazines piled up in his aunt's outhouse, which he dubbed his library. In New York, he graduated from high school, but as the family needed the money, he went to work at local department stores as a packer, earning a dollar an hour. He tried night school, but it wasn't for him, and so in March 1962, he joined the US Army and ended up serving for three years.

As my father tells it, he didn't have his first direct experience with racism until he was twenty-one. The year was 1963 and he was stationed in Texas. One day, on his way from Austin to Fort

Hood with three other soldiers, they decided to stop for a drink at a bar. The one white soldier in the group went ahead of my father to buy his beer. My dad followed him. As soon as he walked in, my father saw the bartender pointing and telling someone to get out. When my father looked behind him, there was no one else there. Shocked, he realized the bartender was shouting at him. He went back to the car.

The other soldiers laughed at him for being so naive. The bar was segregated.

"Where did you think you were going?" one of them asked.

My father felt stunned and humiliated. He thought they considered him to be an arrogant foreigner who needed to be brought down a peg. Until then, his only experience with racism had been subtle or secondhand, reading about it in books.

After leaving the army in 1965, my father was able to use veteran benefits to pay for his tuition at New York City Community College and then Brooklyn College, where he met my mother. However, throughout his studies he still had to work menial jobs to pay for living and other expenses: he repaired cigarette lighters, pushed clothing racks in the Garment District, worked the night shift in a bank, and took a job as a janitor at a pool club. Frequently, he would go up for positions only to be told outright that he wasn't going to be hired due to his race. After graduation, he earned his MBA from Baruch College, another City University of New York institution, and then went to work for the New York City Board of Education. During the Civil Rights era, my father became increasingly political. He had seen his once-thriving Black neighborhood of Bed-Stuy destroyed by the 1964 uprisings that took place after James Powell, a fifteen-year-old Black boy, was shot and killed by police in front of his friends and many other witnesses. These events led to six consecutive days and nights of protests in both Harlem and in his neighborhood.

As a result of events like these, my father began to embrace Afrocentric movements. He joined a cultural and educational center in the neighborhood called the East that had been founded by educators inspired by the Black nationalist and Pan-African movements of the 1960s. The East was a place where you could learn about politics, history, and your roots. My father was also drawn there because of the music. Some of the greatest jazz musicians of the era played at the East, including Pharoah Sanders, who named his 1972 album *Live at the East*. The East had its own newspaper and its own independent school where students were taught the principles of self-determination and Black consciousness. It was one of the first organizations in New York to promote the celebration of Kwanzaa.

Many of the people my parents met at the East had changed their "government" names to African names—and so when my mother became pregnant with my sister and me, they decided to give us West African names. Our parents had traveled to Greece on their babymoon while our mother was pregnant with us. They met two Nigerian men while in Greece during their travels. One of the men's names was Uchechukwu, an Igbo name, meaning "God's will." My parents loved the name and its meaning. They chose to name me Uché for short and added the *accent aigu* on the *e* to ensure people in the US would pronounce my name properly. Oni's name, which means "one born in a sacred place," is a Yoruba name, a language which is spoken in parts of West Africa, including Nigeria. My middle name is Abebe, which is Amharic, from Ethiopia, and my sister's middle name is Jahi, which is Swahili. Even though my parents weren't born in Africa—and we don't know exactly where in West Africa our ancestors trace back to— our parents were intentional about creating a connection to the motherland.

My father's Pan-African politics were key to his sense of identity. The other defining factor for him was being a homeowner. For my dad, as an immigrant, owning a home was the pinnacle of success. As a young boy, he had experienced the deadly 1951 tropical cyclone Hurricane Charlie, which completely destroyed the tiny A-frame house where he lived with his aunt. Like it was for so many immigrants, home ownership was his American dream. As it turned out, that dream was tantalizingly hard to reach. In 1977, when our parents first started looking for a house, they were told they weren't going to be able to qualify for a conventional mortgage despite both having good salaries. Although the 1968 Fair Housing Act had banned housing discrimination based on race, my parents quickly learned they couldn't qualify for Federal Housing Administration–backed mortgages or a homeowners insurance policy because Crown Heights, the predominantly Black neighborhood where they could afford to buy, was considered a risky investment—a remnant of redlining policies. After an extensive search, they learned that the only mortgage given for the area at the time was through Veterans Affairs.

Because my father was a veteran, he was eventually able to get a loan thanks to the Bedford Stuyvesant Restoration Corporation, a nonprofit community development organization. The brainchild of Robert F. Kennedy and the first of its kind in the country, this initiative had been founded to promote and support community development in the area. The same year my parents purchased our childhood home, the Community Reinvestment Act was enacted in an effort to encourage banks to lend to borrowers in lower-income neighborhoods like Crown Heights. Thanks to the Community Reinvestment Act, the community development organization, and my father's status as a veteran, my parents became the first people to get a mortgage through the Bedford Stuyvesant Restoration Corporation. Not only did they have difficulty securing a mortgage but they also were unable to qualify for homeowner's insurance because the neighborhood had been redlined. They spent almost a decade in our home with only a fire insurance policy until they finally were able to qualify for mortgage insurance in the mid-1980s.

The only house that they could afford to buy, however, was nothing short of a wreck. It was a dilapidated four-story brownstone with unstable wood stairs, a collapsing cast iron gate out front, and woodwork covered with countless layers of paint. When our parents first moved into the house, Oni and I were only a few weeks old, and we all had to stay in one room because our parents hadn't had enough time to fix up the rest of the building. At that time, the neighborhood was filled with run-down houses like ours, its streets lined with an array of centuries-old townhouses and brownstones in various states of disrepair. My mother would tell my father, "I can't figure why you chose this block. We used to pass this block as kids and hated it." But my father was set on this block and this house. Our house remained in a constant state of renovation over the next decade, with our father doing most of the work himself on weekends. I rarely saw him without a hammer in hand or a scraper, which he used to remove thickened old paint from the wood moldings. He was always pulling up rotten floorboards or mending the wooden steps or repairing the cracked ceiling.

Our mother worked long hours and we were busy with school, and so the place where we all came together was at the dinner table. Here, our parents talked to us about the difficult experiences that they had and those that were awaiting us in the world. Despite his hard work and smarts, my father was bypassed for promotion multiple times during his career at the Board of Education. Our mother worked in a hospital where most patients were Black, but her bosses and everyone on the board was white. Our parents would talk often about the struggles they faced: being disrespected at work, not getting promotions they deserved, and painful interactions with others. They knew the United States would be a hostile place for my sister and me, but they believed that if we kept our heads down and worked hard enough, we would prevail. We followed their lead. We did the work, got the grades, and went to good schools. We excelled.

Looking back at my parents' heroic efforts to attain home ownership—my dad's tireless work to fix up our house, and their determination to talk to us about racism while still ensuring that we should have every opportunity in life—it breaks my heart that I still learned to feel internalized shame about the block I called home. I didn't understand or know the answers at the time, and it would take many years for me to appreciate how systemic racism in its various forms had negatively impacted every aspect of my parents' life, my life, and my community. It was only as I got older and began to open my eyes that I came to ask the crucial question: Why? Why were there uprisings in my community? Why were the neighborhoods where my classmates lived filled with streets with trees, unlike the barren concrete stretches of my own? Why were so many people from my own community dying from gun violence or crack overdoses or in prison? And why were all the amenities I needed to get ahead in life found in other neighborhoods and not where I lived, among the people I loved and who looked like me?

What I didn't know when I was growing up was that the de facto segregation of neighborhoods in New York I saw all around me was a result of decades of racist federal policies that prevented Black Americans from purchasing houses in certain neighborhoods and, in cities across the country, impacted the health and wealth of generations of Black people. The practice of marking neighborhoods according to the race of its inhabitants dates back to the 1930s, when the federal government decided it wanted to evaluate various residential areas across the country according to their "riskiness" for mortgage lenders. Bureaucrats at the federal Home Owners' Loan Corporation sat down and decided to color-code neighborhoods according to the "danger" posed by borrowers to lenders. Neighborhoods that were considered the highest risk were marked in red—and banks were duly alerted that it was not going to be a good idea to lend money to people in those areas. These redlined areas also happened to be the parts of the country with the highest populations of Black people and other people of color and immigrants. Today, the practice of redlining is considered one of the main reasons that Black communities have been systematically shut out of the wealth-building opportunities of home ownership, concentrating poverty in disinvested neighborhoods that were ringed in red close to a century ago. Our own neighborhood of Crown Heights was redlined, which I know now is the reason why my parents were blocked from obtaining a conventional mortgage.

Redlining wasn't the only racist barrier to housing of the mid-last century. In 1944, the GI Bill offered housing provisions to white veterans while denying them to the more than one million Black veterans who had served in World War II. While nothing in the bill explicitly stated that Black veterans should be exempt from the kinds of low-interest mortgages offered to their white counterparts, the problem was that the loans were not issued by the VA itself. The way it worked was that the VA would cosign the loans, but the banks guaranteed them. This meant that financial institutions could simply turn down mortgages to Black customers with impunity. As a result, white veterans were allowed to benefit from the accumulated wealth of home ownership, passing it down to their children and grandchildren and so on, while the vast majority of Black veterans were not.

For my family, the dream of home ownership became a reality. But what would have happened if we hadn't been able to benefit from the Community Reinvestment Act? What if the Bedford Stuyvesant Restoration Corporation that gave our family the loan hadn't been founded? What if my dad hadn't been a veteran and able to qualify for a mortgage? The window of opportunity for us to obtain that loan was less like a window and more like the eye of a needle—we had simply been fortunate enough to squeeze through it.

The legacy and impact of redlining, the GI Bill, and other racist housing policies have impacted our communities in so many ways, but perhaps the most pernicious has been the effect on health. Without access to loans, redlined neighborhoods fell into further decline, and retailers and other services left or didn't want to provide services in those areas in the first place. This meant the people living in those areas experienced limited access to all kinds of resources and amenities. Research conducted in 2020 by the National Community Reinvestment Coalition, the University of Richmond, and the University of Wisconsin–Milwaukee analyzed 142 metropolitan areas across the country. The researchers took redlined federal maps from the 1930s and then compared them with the economic and health status of residents living in those neighborhoods today. Along with rates of poverty far higher than non-redlined areas, they also found that residents had shorter life spans—sometimes reduced by as much as twenty or thirty years. These same communities had much higher rates of diseases such as asthma, diabetes, hypertension, high cholesterol, kidney disease, obesity, and stroke. Residents in these neighborhoods also suffered higher rates of infant mortality and mental health problems.

Another study, conducted by researchers from the Science

Museum of Virginia, Virginia Commonwealth University, and Portland State University, has found that in 108 urban areas nationwide, formerly redlined neighborhoods were hotter than others, by as much as 13 degrees, due to lack of trees and green spaces. Data from the United States Department of Agriculture tells us that about 23.5 million people live in food deserts in this country—that's around 8.4 percent of the population. This is connected to what's known as "supermarket redlining," which the National Institutes of Health defines as what happens when the big chain supermarkets prefer to locate their stores in the suburbs rather than in low-income, urban neighborhoods where Black and Latinx* people tend to live. We talk about the importance of making good, healthy choices in life, but we often ignore the fact that sometimes there is no choice at all. It's hard to be healthy when you have no place to be outside in nature, when you can't access nutritious food, and when you are subject to pollution and other harmful environmental factors beyond your control.

Today, studies show that your zip code is a much bigger determinant of health outcomes than your DNA. Your zip code determines where you go to school, and your access to decent food, health care, and secure, affordable housing. It affects the kind of jobs and transportation that are available to you, all of which are major determinants in health outcomes. It has affected whether the COVID-19 vaccine will be available to you, with Black and

---

* I have chosen *Latinx* to describe people of Latin American heritage because it is a more inclusive and gender-free alternative to *Latino* or *Latina*.

Latinx communities experiencing a disproportionate lack of access when vaccines were first rolled out, which some have described as "vaccine redlining."

At this point in our nation's history, we have a clearer idea about how racism has harmed the health and well-being of Black people in this country. We know that Black men have the shortest life expectancy, that Black women are more likely to die in child-birth than any other group, and that Black babies are more likely to be born prematurely and underweight. But the problem doesn't lie inherently in us—in our DNA—as I had been made to believe as a child. Studies show that people like my father, coming to the US from the African diaspora, can have excellent health outcomes when they arrive in this country, but for the second generation of their families those outcomes decline, becoming comparable to Black Americans whose enslaved ancestors were brought here in chains. Exposure to racism—and the cumulative trauma caused by lack of access to stable housing, education, resources, and opportunity—has a measurable, deleterious effect on health.

As a child and young person in Brooklyn, I could see the impact of these systemic problems all around me, in the drugs that were destroying the health of my neighbor, in the shootings that imper-iled our neighbors' and our own lives, in the services that we lacked close by simply because of the zip code where we lived. I could see the symptoms, I just couldn't name the disease.

THREE

Everything We Lost

Our mother was a remarkably vibrant and athletic woman. She regularly ran twenty miles a week, a habit she had first picked up in medical school to calm her frazzled nerves. After Oni and I were born, she began squeezing her daily run into the very early mornings before we got up for school and she had to go to work. I can remember from a young age lying in bed, still half-asleep, hearing her getting ready to go out. She'd always come into our room before she left, kissing us goodbye as we dozed back off to sleep. In winter, when the nights were longer, she'd often drive to our nearest green space, Prospect Park, because it wasn't safe to run from home, and complete the more than three-mile loop of the park. She was a petite woman and I worried often about her safety while she was gone on those dark mornings, feeling a real sense of relief when I'd finally hear her key open the front door.

In her younger years, she had run marathons, and even once won as the first woman to cross the finish line. And although after having twins, she gave up running very long distances, she'd still regularly compete in 5K and 10K races in Prospect Park and in Manhattan's Central Park. As children, we loved to watch our mother race. She had such a delicate frame, yet she had real power and speed when she ran, often crossing the finish line ahead of most of the other runners in her age group. She had experienced her own share of racism and sexism while running, with white male runners spitting at her and trash-talking to try unsuccessfully to psych her out. Despite these unpleasant experiences, she encouraged Oni and me to join her in her passion, and I ran my first race with her when I was only six years old. It was a family race in Prospect Park. She ran alongside me the whole way, cheering me on. A picture of us running together was even published in one of the local Brooklyn papers.

As Oni and I got older and entered our preteens, we joined the New York Road Runners club and began competing with her. Even when we were teenagers and she was in her forties, our mother always crossed the line before us—she was unstoppable. Then she would wait for us there, cheering us on.

"Okay, sister, lookin' good!" she'd shout. She often called us "sister" because she wouldn't have to figure out which of our names to call first.

After we crossed the line, she'd run to give us a hug or congratulate us on our times. Thanks to her, we learned to appreciate the sheer endorphin rush that comes from accomplishing a goal that one has set for oneself.

Our mother also taught us about the health benefits of spending time in nature. Besides Prospect Park, where she went for her daily runs, one of her favorite places was the Brooklyn Botanic Garden, about a twenty-five-minute walk from our home. Planted with flowering cherry trees, water lily ponds, and rose gardens, the Botanic Garden was the place where she would take us for regular strolls, pointing out the many varieties of flowers, plants, and trees as she went. Our mother always seemed happy when she was walking in the garden, as if this were a place where she could shed some of the pressures of her daily life, losing herself in the beauty of her surroundings. There was an educational program at the garden for children, and so our mother signed us up so we could learn how to grow vegetables. We planted seeds, nurturing them into seedlings, feeding them with water and compost, and eventually harvesting our own crops. Inspired by our efforts, our mother decided we needed a vegetable patch at home. Long before Michelle Obama dug up the White House lawn to plant vegetables, our mother took a shovel to our backyard so we could have regular crops of potatoes, carrots, corn, and broccoli to eat for dinner.

By the time Oni and I left home to go to Harvard University to study premed, we just assumed that our mother was invincible. It never occurred to us that someone as physically strong, energetic, and with such a healthy lifestyle could get sick. She had poured every ounce of herself into helping us to grow into self-assured young women who would make even better choices in life than she had. Taking care of yourself, feeding your mind and your body, focusing on your education: these were the priorities in our family. She coached us through our college applications; took us to visit Harvard's campus so that when we arrived there for our freshman year, we already felt at home. There was never any question for us that we would do anything else but shape our own paths guided by her constant love and support. That first year away from home, we began finding our feet as we lived in dorms and navigated coursework and a new social life. We still spoke with our mother on the phone every day, but we were eighteen years old, beginning to separate from her, forging our own identities.

Her illness interrupted all of that. The first time I remember noticing any change was during a 10K race. It was the summer of 1996, between our freshman and sophomore year. Oni and I had signed up to race with our mother in Central Park. Usually, we would expect her to be ahead of us, but this particular day, I remember looking over my shoulder and thinking, "Where is she?" When she came in a good few minutes after we crossed the finish line, I asked her if she was okay.

"I don't know what happened," she replied between deep breaths. She was bent over with her hands on her hips and head down. "I just feel really tired."

On the way home, our mother confided to Oni and me that she had been feeling under the weather for a while. She had been to her physician; they had done blood work and believed she had a vitamin B_{12} deficiency because her red blood cells were so big. When you don't have enough vitamin B_{12}, your bone marrow makes abnormally large red blood cells. She was getting B_{12} shots, but they didn't seem to be helping. Eventually, her doctors did a more thorough workup, including a bone marrow biopsy. This took several weeks. I remember telling her to please keep us posted about the results, and soon after that we returned for our second year at Harvard.

One day, when we were back in Boston and two months into our sophomore year, we got a call from our mother's sister, Auntie Joanie. She lived in the Boston area and had always been like a second mother to us. We would see her often, so it wasn't unusual for her to call and come over to visit. Aunt Joanie and our mother were close, even though Joanie, who was about seven inches taller than her big sister, was eight years younger. When I saw our aunt's face as she walked into our dormitory that day, I knew it was bad news—her usual cheery disposition was gone, and instead she looked distraught, her eyes somehow sunken into her features. We walked out to the courtyard outside our dorm, which over-looked the Charles River. It was a slightly chilly fall day, the clouds overhead casting dark shadows across the silvery water. As she told us about our mother's diagnosis, all three of us started to cry. I realized that our mother must have sent her sister to tell us be-cause she couldn't bear to do it herself. I remember dropping to my knees on the ground and sobbing.

Our mother had been diagnosed with acute myelogenous leu-kemia (AML), a type of blood cancer. Her doctors gave her two to three months to live. The chemotherapy treatments started right away. Oni and I spent that year traveling back and forth between Boston and New York, on buses, trains, and airplanes, while our mother was in and out of the hospital. In many ways, being a phy-sician was the hardest part of her illness, because she knew ex-actly what was taking place in her body. I remember sitting next to her hospital bed catching up on college work when the medical team would make rounds, crowding around her, delivering updates on lab tests or bone marrow results, our mother looking frail and tiny by comparison. My mother's cancer taught me that to be a patient is one of the most vulnerable experiences you can have as a human being. To put your care, your health, your life into the hands of someone else takes enormous courage and strength. When she got sick, she had to put her trust in others. That shift in roles, from the person who always cared for others to the person who had to rely on others for that care, must have been so painful for her.

Yet despite the odds, she told us that she would beat the disease, that she would endure the harsh chemotherapy side effects, infections, and sheer pain and discomfort to do so. That she was a fighter.

There are multiple risk factors for AML, and although the official list doesn't include racism, I can't help but wonder about the many ways systemic racism may have contributed to my mother's increased susceptibility to the disease. Not long after her diagnosis, she came up to Boston for a second opinion at the Dana-Farber Cancer Institute, one of the leading cancer centers in the country, if not the world. Our father made the four-hour drive from NYC with our mother resting in the back seat of our family's boxy burgundy Volvo. I remember him referring to her as "precious cargo" when they arrived safely with us in Cambridge. At that point, she had lost considerable weight; she couldn't have been more than one hundred pounds. Her hair had fallen out in clumps from the chemotherapy, and she wore a thick wool hat over her newly smooth, brown bald head. She was wrapped in homemade quilts made by a family friend to keep her warm. After her visit with the oncologist, she told us that the doctor who had looked at her karyotype—a picture of the chromosomes at the cellular level—said it seemed to him as if she had been exposed to high doses of radiation at some point in her life, which would have increased her risk for her type of cancer.

At the time, I didn't think to ask how this might have been possible. I was too distraught and worried about her to think much about anything else. Since that time, I've come to understand that my mother may well have been exposed to radiation as a child or perhaps even in utero. Today, there are four designated "Superfund" sites in New York City, locations that the Environmental Protection Agency has marked as polluted by hazardous waste and in need of cleanup. Two of the four sites are radioactive dumping grounds: one of these is in Brooklyn and one is on the Brooklyn-Queens border, both in Black and Latinx communities where my mother lived. Multiple studies show that people who reside in predominantly low-income communities of the kind my mother grew up in have much higher exposure to toxic environmental contaminants in general, which in turn can lead to higher instances of cancer.

We also know that these high rates are compounded by the fact that Black patients often have delayed cancer diagnoses due to lack of access to health care and lack of quality, culturally responsive care. By the time my mother's leukemia was caught, it was already extremely advanced and therefore much more difficult to treat. When her oncologists looked back at her blood work, they could see that her red blood cells had been enlarged for a while, at least one to two years. But this key indicator for her disease wasn't picked up by her primary care physician in Brooklyn, who had told her at first, when her symptoms began, that she needed to take vitamin B_{12} for a deficiency. Certain cancers have a high chance of cure if they are detected at any early stage and adequately treated, but if these cancers aren't detected early, then the chance of mortality becomes much higher.

There may have been additional factors that increased the degree to which the disease ripped through my mother's body with such ferocity. As a physician herself, she had more access to medical information and quality care than most people. She was treated by some of the best physicians in New York at the time and kept a close eye on the care she received. But what if the treatment she received wasn't the kind she really needed? Recent studies point to the continued overrepresentation of white patients in clinical oncology trials, which may be another reason for the unfavorable outcomes we see for Black cancer patients. For decades, Black patients have been disproportionately underrepresented in cancer studies, the results of which are generally assumed to be applicable to everyone. But how can we be certain of universal applicability if Black people are excluded from trials in the first place?

Aging is another key risk factor in my mother's disease. Although people can develop AML at all ages, the risk increases substantially as someone gets older. My mother was in the prime of her life, in her midforties, when she was struck down by AML. But what if the cells in her relatively young body had gone through an accelerated aging process due to her life experiences as a Black woman? Studies have shown that the higher levels of stress to which Black people are subjected on a day-to-day basis due to racism can, in turn, cause our cells to divide and deteriorate, accelerating the body's aging process. This phenomenon has been dubbed "weathering" or "premature aging" by public health researcher Dr. Arline Geronimus, who first noted the effects of increased stress on the health of pregnant teenagers in Black and Latinx communities in New Jersey when compared with their white counterparts. Geronimus chose the term *weathering*—the process of a rock being worn down by long exposure to atmospheric elements—to deliberately evoke the erosion of youth due to the cumulative "drip, drip, drip" effect of racism in the lives of Black and Latinx people.

Like anyone Black in the United States, our mother had experienced the excruciating pain of that slow and constant drip firsthand. Growing up in poverty, she had been forced to constantly move to different schools and apartments due to housing insecurity, and she never knew if there would be enough food on the table. She was the first person in her family to go to college, the first to have a professional career, navigating a demanding medical career without mentorship or support. The culture of medicine is unforgiving; you have to give so much of yourself—and to add to that, she was working in an underserved area, in an under-resourced hospital, seeing people with chronic medical problems resulting from the same lack of housing and food stability she had experienced as a child. On top of this, there was the everyday discrimination she experienced as a matter of course. I can remember the time Oni and I watched in horror as a CVS pharmacy security guard accused our mother of stealing something from the store and demanded she open her bag. Our always firm and confident mother was suddenly flustered, embarrassed, made vulnerable by this awful stranger who somehow held power over her, and by extension us. We were furious and scared, clinging to her as she opened her purse. Another time, she came home shaken and crying. When we asked what had happened, she told us she had parked a little too close to a bus stop and when a police officer asked her to move, she hadn't moved fast enough for his liking, and so he had asked her to get out of the car and then pushed her up against it.

People often talk about "going to war" with cancer or "the fight" to combat the disease, but we hear less about how the "war" and "fight" a person endures before they get visibly sick may have contributed to a physical diminishment of the body. And our mother is far from an outlier. Today, the National Cancer Institute's database shows that Black patients with AML have a 12 percent increased risk for mortality compared with white patients who have the disease, but we will need far more studies that include Black people before we truly understand why. To this day, I wonder whether our mother might have lived longer had she not been Black in America. Although we'll never know for certain, what we do know is that the ongoing impact of racism on Black bodies continues to leave untold loss in its wake.

<hr />

As the weeks passed after her diagnosis, our mother's chemotherapy treatments became more intense. Incredibly, her brother, my uncle Tyrone, turned out to be a bone marrow match. The goal was to clean out her bone marrow with chemotherapy and then replace it with my uncle's healthy bone marrow cells. She never went into remission from the chemotherapy, however. The bone marrow transplant was unable to happen and her health continued to worsen. We began to face the fact that she might never get better.

We had some tough but honest conversations during that time, some in person, others on the phone. One night during my sophomore year, as my roommates went out to parties, I stayed in my room, on the phone with my mother back in Brooklyn, lying on the floor, looking up at the ceiling.

"Mommy?" I asked softly.

"Yes," she replied.

I paused, then blurted out, "What are some things that I should know for the future, things that we won't be able to talk about later?"

I could hear her inhale deeply.

"You need to take care of yourself," she told me. "Make sure you always put yourself first. Always. Even when you have your babies, you put yourself first."

In the depths of her illness, my mother was sending me a clear message about the importance of my own physical and mental health. Despite the self-care she had practiced—her daily morning runs and the afternoons walking in the Brooklyn Botanic Garden or tending her vegetable patch—she had spent so much of her life giving to others: her children, spouse, extended family, mentees, and her community. I have wondered since if she was also telling me that she regretted not making more time for herself, that she didn't want me to make the same mistake.

A few days after that conversation, I overheard her talking to my aunt on the phone.

"Do you know my baby asked me if we could talk about some of the things that she won't be able to talk to me about later? I was so proud of her. I was so proud of my baby for having the strength to ask me."

As I listened to those words, I did feel proud of myself, but also scared about what the future would bring. By having that conversation that night, she and I had confronted the fact that she was going to die, and soon. The chemotherapy wasn't working. Her kind of leukemia was so resistant that the cancer never went into remission. Then she developed a devastating fungal infection in her lungs because the chemotherapy had so suppressed her immune system.

One day she told me, "I'm so tired, and I don't want to do this anymore."

"You don't have to do it anymore, Mommy," I said.

At that moment, any hold I had on her, I released it. I was accepting her death. That's true love. True love was letting her go in peace, because the chemotherapy treatments were making her sick. She made it until July 5, 1997, outlasting the doctors' prognoses by several months. Oni and I were home from college for the summer. I was doing a summer research program at NYU School of Medicine and Oni had taken an internship at AT&T in New Jersey. Our mother had begun having a lot of trouble breathing at home due to her lung infection. We moved her to the hospital so she could start receiving palliative care. The morning of the fifth, we visited her early in the day. She was in a small room with a single bed and two chairs, light falling on her face through double windows, a morphine drip at her side that she could administer herself with a small button. She seemed to be sleeping, as if she were finally comfortable. Our father explained that the doctor had told him that she didn't have much time left.

That day, Oni and I had tickets to a concert at Jones Beach that we had bought many months ago. The lineup included the singer-songwriter Erykah Badu, one of our favorites, and it was taking place about an hour's drive from the hospital. We didn't know if we should go, but our father insisted.

"You should go to the concert," he told us. "She'd want you to go, to be enjoying yourself."

And so, we went. There was so much traffic getting out of there and coming back—we both knew that there was a chance that she would pass while we were gone. The concert took place in an outdoor amphitheater on the water. It was a hot day, but the breeze from the ocean felt like a balm. Losing ourselves in the large crowd, we danced along to the eclectic mix of soul, hip-hop, and funk artists: Badu but also Cypress Hill, George Clinton and the P-Funk All Stars, the Roots, and Foxy Brown.

After the concert, we drove back to the hospital, and as we pulled into the parking lot, one of the nurses was leaving and rolled down her window.

"I'm so sorry . . ." she cried out.

This was how we learned. We went up to our mother's room, and she was there, lying in her bed. Our aunt had surrounded her body with cool white towels, and only her thin, gaunt face peeked through, looking finally at peace. Our dad had been at her bedside when she died; she hadn't been alone. She looked like she might have been sleeping, her eyelids closed. I kissed her forehead gently; held her hand, which was still warm. I told her I loved her. Oni did the same. I remember feeling such incredible sadness but also relief that she was at peace.

Our mother hadn't wanted a funeral; she'd wanted to be cremated. Her memorial service was held in an old Victorian mansion in our neighborhood in Bed-Stuy that was owned by family friends who rented out the bottom floors for events. The building had been meticulously restored over a number of years, a gorgeous, grand space that was still very intimate. Our mother had loved classical music and so there was a string quartet playing downstairs as people arrived. Her siblings and their children, her nieces and nephews, her current and former colleagues, family friends, mentees, even patients of hers that she had treated over the years were there. Upstairs in the living room there was a grand piano and we gathered around it, everyone sharing memories of her, people speaking to how much she was loved and admired, her kindness, her integrity. Jitu Weusi, one of the founders of the East, the Pan-African organization to which my mother and father belonged, spoke about her community-mindedness, her determination to address health inequities in our city. One of her colleagues, a nephrologist, spoke about how our mother was friends with everyone at the hospital, from the clerks to the chairs of the departments. I had brought a framed photo of her to place on the piano, but I couldn't let it go, and so instead I held it in my arms tightly, like I was holding on to her.

She had given us instructions from her hospital bed, telling us that she wanted her ashes scattered in her two favorite places, Prospect Park and the Brooklyn Botanic Garden. One of our uncles, Ricky, who looked the most like our mother of all her siblings and was closest to her in age, helped us to lay her to rest. He was a long-distance runner like our mother, and so one early morning he took her ashes and ran the circuit of Prospect Park, as she had done so many times in her life, scattering every now and then a small handful of her ashes as he ran. Later that same morning, we took the rest of the ashes to the Botanic Garden, to her favorite spot in the Japanese Hill-and-Pond Garden, one of the most serene places in the city, shaded with maple and pine trees. There, standing on a small wooden bridge, we cast her ashes out on the water. In quiet tones, I thanked her—for her love, her affection, for being an inspiration, and for being the best mother I could have asked for, even if for only nineteen years of my life. The park had been the place where she went to run, but the Botanic Garden had been her oasis, the place where she could finally be still.

FOUR

All the Things They Didn't Teach Me

In the immediate aftermath of our mother's death, I remember waking up in the mornings and feeling like my head was too heavy to pick up off the pillow. My sense of dread at having to confront the world without her was palpable; I felt nauseated, my entire body heavy. Oni and I had stayed in New York City to complete our summer research programs. I went back to the dorms at NYU School of Medicine and Oni continued living at home. The only reason I didn't huddle in bed in those early days was because I knew that my research was waiting for me. My research project was in an oncology lab, so I had the benefit of knowing I was making some small contribution to cancer research. This, together with my kind and sympathetic new friends from the research program, helped give me the impetus to get out of bed every morning. It was a tough summer, but I was grateful to have meaningful work, to be close to my sister and father, and the places I associated with our mother. I cried a lot, almost every day. Talking to

Oni gave me some relief, but she was going through her own grieving process and could only support me so much.

Our mother, being who she was, had left us with clear instructions for what to do after she was gone. As we helped our father to clear out her things, we found a handwritten letter under her mattress addressed to us. In the letter, she tenderly instructed us to take care of each other and go on to medical school. Just as she had suggested, we had begun seeing a grief counselor even before her death to help us manage our inevitable loss. And in September, we returned to Cambridge and to our studies. Despite the heavy weight of how much I missed her—which at times I felt in every fiber of my being—I actually did my best academic work in those last two years of college. I found solace in my studies, especially my premed classes. I did not feel like socializing much with my peers, who seemed so carefree in comparison to the heaviness I felt as I mourned my mother's death, so I spent a lot of time those last two years with Oni in the library, our noses in our textbooks.

Again, acting on our mother's instructions, we decided to delay entry into medical school. Although she had told us firmly that she didn't want us to take time off during college, she did feel it was important for us to have a break from our education *after* we graduated.

"Promise me you'll take time off before you start medical school," she had insisted from her hospital bed. "To get your bearings together."

"Get my bearings together" was one of my mother's favorite expressions. When she felt overwhelmed by life, she would say, "I have to get my bearings together," which meant she needed some time to herself. I think she worried that by the time we graduated, we would be emotionally drained and not in a good place mentally and psychologically to start medical school. I'm grateful to my mother for many reasons, but that she would in her own time of need make sure that her daughters were going to take care of their own selves means a great deal to me.

After graduation, following our mother's advice, both Oni and I applied to teach at independent schools in different parts of the country: I got a job at a private school in Chicago, and Oni left for a teaching position in Northern Virginia. My year in Chicago was a huge eye-opener: this was the first time that I'd lived anywhere without Oni. I had my first apartment, my first car, and first job—a lot of firsts that were difficult to experience on my own. The high school where I taught biology and chemistry had mostly students from white, very affluent backgrounds. Even though the school reminded me very much of where we had attended junior high school, I felt like I was moving through foreign waters now as a teacher, wading out of my depth. Ever since I had been a baby, my mother had been my anchor. She had chosen to be a mother—she and my father had tried several times to get pregnant before she got pregnant with us. Oni and I had always felt loved and grounded by our attachment to her. There were so many times when I was in Chicago that I just wanted to pick up the phone and call her, to hear her voice, for her to comfort me. Without her, I was adrift.

The following year, Oni started her first semester at Harvard Medical School, but I decided I wanted to take another year to continue to get my bearings together. I applied for a job at a health-care advocacy organization called Health Care for All in Boston, where I ended up working on a tobacco tax campaign. I visited state representatives at the statehouse to lobby for the tax, the revenue of which would go toward funding health insurance for uninsured and underinsured people in Massachusetts. I also learned a lot about how public policy can improve health outcomes. I enjoyed the experience, but I always knew that I would follow my mother's path to medical school.

In the fall of 2001, at the age of twenty-three, I took my place as a student at Harvard Medical School, or HMS, as we always called it. My time off between college and medical school in Chicago and Boston had been a welcome respite from the high expectations of academia, and now I was more than ready for medical school. I remember the first day at HMS, I bumped into Dr. Alvin Poussaint, the smiling, well-dressed associate dean of diversity and multicultural affairs. Dr. Poussaint was a legend. He had been at HMS since the 1960s, before my mother was even a student there, and had founded the Office of Recruitment and Multicultural Affairs in 1969. Under Dr. Poussaint's leadership, diversity initiatives flourished, making HMS one of the medical schools with the largest percentage of historically excluded students in the country. With open arms, Dr. Poussaint welcomed me to medical school. During our conversation, he fondly recalled my mother and shared that he was quite pleased to have both my sister and me at HMS to continue our mother's legacy. That day at HMS, I knew exactly where I was supposed to be. Knowing that my mother had spent time there was incredibly meaningful to me: I was finally fulfilling her dreams.

Oni and I found an apartment together off campus in the Fields

Corner area of Dorchester, a diverse working- and middle-class neighborhood that reminded us of where we had grown up in Brooklyn. Classes were a short drive away, and Oni and I shared our mother's old burgundy Volvo sedan. We fell into a routine of driving to classes together, then we would meet up for lunchtime talks at school to take advantage of the free lunches, and to hang out with the staff in the Office of Recruitment and Multicultural Affairs. Dr. Poussaint always seemed to have time to counsel us and hear about our latest news, and his office gave us a place to call home at HMS. While our mother was one of only a handful of Black students in her time, ours was a much larger cohort, and we were able to feel supported rather than singled out. The campus in the fall was so beautiful, the trees lining the main quad turning bright orange and rust brown with crisp blue skies overhead. I began a new ritual of running along the Charles River, training for the New York City Marathon, which I ran twice while at medical school. Running became an escape for me, just as it had been for my mother. I found the pounding of my feet under me to be meditative, and I think it helped me in my ongoing journey through grief.

Although you might expect the academic load at a top-tier medical school to be onerous, it was actually quite manageable. The first two years at HMS we were graded using a pass-fail system, which made learning more enjoyable than in college, where we received letter grades and were graded on a curve, which is why students who attend HMS often joke that the hardest part about HMS is getting in. I was a diligent student, eager to get back into study mode after taking time off, hurrying to classes through the atrium of the main teaching building, a large open space with couches where students gather to socialize. I was hungry to learn all the things that I thought I was supposed to learn to become a skilled and competent physician, to be given the keys to a greater understanding of the human body, its functions, its frailties, and how to make things better.

Yet despite the sterling efforts of Dr. Poussaint and his office to admit and retain Black, Latinx, and Indigenous students, the same commitment to diversity was not reflected in the faculty or the curriculum in the early 2000s. Looking back, I can see there were stunning omissions and flaws in my education. During my four years at HMS, I don't remember anyone ever talking about racial health inequities in medicine; there was never any conversation about the glaring discrepancy in outcomes between Black and white patients, or the nuances of how to competently care for patients of different racial and ethnic backgrounds. Our professors were overwhelmingly white men; I could count the number of Black faculty members on one hand. From our instructors, we learned to see the world through what was considered an entirely "scientific, objective, and evidence-based" lens. These men were immensely confident, seemingly competent authorities on their subjects. It was not our job to doubt them, it was our job to absorb everything they told us, from the Krebs cycle, a critical metabolic pathway in the cells of organisms that use oxygen, to the Frank-Starling curve, a mechanism in the heart that relates to the filling of ventricles to the blood pumped out of the heart into the body.

"This is how this process works," we were told. "We know this because of the landmark study published in *The New England Journal of Medicine.*"

The information imparted to us in the classrooms and on the wards was presented as "factual data" and "research-driven" without any sociopolitical context.

I now realize that this so-called objectivity was anything but.

———

A lot of the time, it wasn't as much a case of what our professors were teaching us as what they were leaving out. No one ever spoke about the fact that Black people had been forced and coerced into enduring often-violent medical or surgical interventions in the name of scientific progress in the country, starting when they were first kidnapped from West Africa and trafficked to the British colony of Virginia in 1619. We know that during the time of slavery, enslaved people were routinely used for medical observation and experimentation, and these practices were allowed to continue into the era of Reconstruction and Jim Crow. Both Northern and Southern medical schools, including HMS and the Universities of Maryland, Pennsylvania, and Virginia even employed what they called "resurrectionists," or grave robbers, to dig up the recently deceased from Black cemeteries to use for education and research. Many of them had been enslaved when they were alive. Such exploitation of Black people for the purposes of medical education is well documented—and yet any discussion of it was absent from our curriculum at HMS in the early 2000s.

In histology class, we studied tissues and their structure under the microscope using HeLa cells to help us understand what normal tissue looks like and how it works, in order to help us recognize different diseases. It wasn't until I was a practicing physician that I learned about the woman to whom those cells had belonged, after the publication of Rebecca Skloot's book, *The Immortal Life of Henrietta Lacks*, which went on to sell more than 2.5 million copies and eventually became an HBO film produced by Oprah Winfrey. As Skloot describes, Henrietta Lacks was a thirty-one-year-old Black woman from impoverished Baltimore when, in 1950, she sought care at the Johns Hopkins Hospital for abdominal pain and was diagnosed with advanced cervical cancer shortly thereafter. During radiation treatment, doctors removed two samples of cervical tissue from her body without her knowledge or consent. She died only ten months later, yet her stolen cells were immortalized and have been used for the past seventy years in medical studies, some of which have resulted in groundbreaking discoveries and innovations, including in HPV and polio vaccine development. (Of note, Skloot worked closely with Henrietta's youngest daughter, Deborah Lacks, for almost ten years researching the book; however, some family members, including Lacks's oldest son, Lawrence, felt Skloot failed to capture their mother's grace and misrepresented the family in the book.) Medical students study Lacks's cells in histology classes to this day, and many dozens of pharmaceutical companies continue to profit from them, with Lacks receiving only belated acknowledgment and without her family having received any financial compensation for decades for the use of their loved one's cells. When I finally learned that "HeLa" stood for Henrietta Lacks, I was thirty-three years old. I felt betrayed by my education—and sick to my stomach.

Similarly, in our gynecology classes, we learned about the vaginal speculum, the medical tool used to examine and dilate a woman's vagina to examine the cervix. But no one ever taught us that Dr. J. Marion Sims, the so-called father of modern gynecology, had invented the tool while conducting research on enslaved Black women, upon whom he also performed excruciatingly painful surgeries without their consent—and without anesthetic. These women, Anarcha, Betsy, and Lucy, were living on different plantations in Alabama in the 1840s when they developed a medical condition brought on by childbirth that caused them to no longer have control of their bladders and bowels. Their enslavers "leased" them to Sims so that he could experiment on the women, while also forcing them to serve as nurses in his clinic and as domestic workers in his household. On Anarcha alone, Sims performed thirty painful surgical procedures. Despite these horrific acts, or perhaps because of them, Sims went on to become the president of the American Medical Association in 1876. In 1880, he became president of the American Gynecological Society. There are over a half dozen statues of Sims in this country, including one in Central Park that was finally removed in 2018, and that I had been walking past unknowingly since I was a young girl.

At medical school we were taught how to diagnose and treat sexually transmitted infections, but no one uttered a word about the Black men who unwittingly submitted to the US Public Health Service's Tuskegee Study of Untreated Syphilis in the Negro Male, which was conducted for four long decades, from 1932 to 1972. The sole purpose of the study was to observe the natural course of untreated syphilis in impoverished Black sharecroppers from rural Alabama, but the many hundreds of Black men who participated in the study were not informed of its objectives and instead were told that they were being treated for "bad blood." The study's racist premise presumed that there were significant differences in how syphilis affected Black and white people. Specifically the belief that because Black people had primitive nervous systems (brains), syphilis was more likely to impact white people's nervous systems and Black people's cardiovascular systems. Of course, there were no white participants. The study only enrolled Black participants. Even in 1947, when effective treatments for syphilis, including penicillin, became available, the disease was allowed to progress untreated in the participants, causing them to needlessly suffer in the name of medical progress.

Such experiments and interventions that were carried out on Black Americans have gone on to create what has often been described as "institutional distrust"—in which Black people are perceived to be reluctant to interact with a medical system that has historically perpetrated abuses upon them. However, this term pathologizes and places the blame on Black people. Instead, this phenomenon is better described as "institutional *untrustworthiness*," whereby institutions have shown themselves to be untrustworthy to our communities thanks to a litany of abuses and mistreatment enacted against Black Americans by the healthcare system. You might have thought that the concept of institutional untrustworthiness as well as the stories of Henrietta

Lacks, Anarcha, Betsy, Lucy, and the men of the Tuskegee Study might have warranted inclusion in our education. But they were nowhere in sight.

Although I wasn't always aware of it at the time, subtle and sometimes not-so-subtle racism permeated my medical school education. In the classroom, a lot of time was spent on teaching us about diagnosis, obviously an important skill for any aspiring physician. As a keen and willing student, I recognized readily that accurate diagnosis is vital; a misdiagnosis could cost someone their health and even their life. In our lectures and small groups, we were given various standard patterns and formulas that were supposed to aid us in more easily recognizing symptoms and identifying their causes. These aids were shortcuts, helping us to diagnose with greater efficiency, and they are used widely. But as I later came to understand, they were also embedded with bias.

Throughout our medical school education, we learned that there were different standards of normal for different patients, and that, along with age and gender, race was one of the principal factors we should consider when assessing a patient. When diagnosing kidney dysfunction, for example, we were taught that Black patients had higher normal kidney function than non-Black patients, based on the racist presumption that Black people have a higher amount of muscle mass. Much later in my career I learned that this particular race-based testing has horrifically led to kidney function being underestimated in Black patients, leaving them less likely to receive the specialty kidney care they need or being excluded from the kidney transplant waitlist because their kidney function may appear normal.

The idea that Black people are biologically different from white people—and even inferior—and therefore need to be treated differently can be traced all the way back to slavery, when white Southern enslavers, challenged by the growing abolitionist movement to dismantle servitude, turned to medical professionals to help perpetuate the lie that people of African descent belonged to a completely different species than white Europeans. If these men could medically "prove" that Black people were "less than human," they could argue that it was in fact the right and moral thing to do to continue to enslave them. Enslavers found willing collaborators in the medical profession, including one Dr. Charles Caldwell, founder of the University of Louisville. After traveling to France in the 1820s, Caldwell learned about the latest medical craze in Europe, phrenology. Returning to the United States, he became one of this country's leading proponents of pseudoscience, which posits that the shape of someone's head is the best predictor of that person's ability and talents. Caldwell, who believed that there were four species of humans—Caucasian, Mongolian, American Indian, and African—wrote popular and influential papers that insisted that enslaved Africans had bumps on the back of their heads that correlated with them being "tameable," and "in need of a master." Phrenology has long since been debunked, and yet medical schools up until recently still taught our medical students in ways that dangerously suggest that Black patients are biologically different, and even inferior.

We can see the same racist histories when we look at pulmonary function tests (noninvasive tests to show how well the lungs are working). At medical school, we'd learned what the test would look like for someone with emphysema, chronic obstructive pulmonary disease, or pulmonary fibrosis, but we'd also learned what the test was going to look like for a Black patient versus a white patient. As with kidney function, race-corrected pulmonary function tests can favor white patients for lung transplants earlier in the course of their disease over Black patients, creating dangerous inequities in outcomes. When I was a student, tables containing these shortcuts to diagnosis were repeated in lectures, in textbooks, and across the scientific literature, but no one ever taught us their racist origins. In fact, the pulmonary function test dates back to the 1850s when a plantation physician from Louisiana, Dr. Samuel Cartwright, insisted that he had proved that Black people had a lesser lung capacity than white people. According to Cartwright, the only cure for this deficit was "forced labor." This was not his only outrageous claim in the name of science—he also believed that Black people who fled their masters were suffering from a mental illness he dubbed "drapetomania." Yet Cartwright's legacy lives on. The spirometer, a device we still use to measure pulmonary function in patients, was actually invented by none other than Cartwright—and modern versions of the device still include software that adjusts for the assumption that Black people have lesser lung capacity than white people.

Throughout history, eminent white physicians whose names live on in the annals and who are celebrated with statues and portraits in our universities have been responsible for originating and perpetuating fallacies about Black people that the medical profession has yet to shake off. In the 1820s, Dr. Thomas Hamilton, a physician from Georgia, claimed to have proved that Black people had thicker skin than white people and therefore were less susceptible to pain. His experiments were conducted on an enslaved man named John Brown, who had no choice but to endure Hamilton's torturous interventions, which involved repeated blistering of the skin. Hamilton's false claims went on to be used by slaveholders to argue that Black people were well suited to enslavement due to their ability to tolerate pain. You might hope that modern medicine would have broken free from such a toxic myth. Instead, according to a paper published in 2016, a survey of white medical students and residents found that around a third of those surveyed still believe that Black and white people have biological differences, that Black people feel less pain than white people, and that Black people have thicker skin. These students and residents were also more likely to suggest inadequate doses of pain medication for Black patients due to such erroneous beliefs.

Like me, generations of medical students were never taught *why* racial distinctions were being made in diagnosis. No one ever discussed with us *why* a Black person might have kidney malfunction or lungs that were damaged, the historical, societal, and environmental factors that might have contributed to his or her health challenges. There was no conversation about how Black Americans have been historically oppressed and denied access to basic needs across centuries. We didn't learn about how, after emancipation, the formerly enslaved were denied the land and livestock they had been promised, which led to them being deprived of a means of survival, forcing them into unhealthy living conditions that disproportionately exposed them to disease, injury, and other forms of physical suffering, without access to adequate medical care. Four hundred years after slavery, we know that inequities in housing, employment, health care, and education persist, continuing to affect health outcomes, and hospitals serving our populations are direly underfunded. And so, when we teach our medical students about the differences in lung or kidney function between Black and white patients, we need to also talk about structural inequities, like systemic racism, that influence the social determinants of health, including environmental exposures, job opportunities, and lack of access to health care. If we allow students to erroneously believe that the differences between Black and white patients are purely genetic or biological, as medical school instructors did in the past century and even now, then we will continue to perpetrate a racist lie.

Throughout my medical education, differences between Black and white patients were passed off as information, as data, as the objective truth. No one made the point that using race as an aid in diagnosis might lead to bias and stereotyping, which in turn could lead to misdiagnosis, thereby harming Black patients. Or perhaps most important, no one stated that race is, after all, a social construct invented during colonial times with no basis in science or genetic fact in the first place. As a student, I'd write everything down in my notebook, barely questioning the underlying assumptions. I was still so naive, studying at one of the best medical schools in the world. Surely the instructors behind the lectern knew what they were talking about. I duly absorbed the message that people of different racial backgrounds have different criteria for what are considered normal laboratory values and that the reason for this was likely biological. The message was clear. We, Black people, had impaired functioning *because of our race.* Whereas the more accurate statement would be that oftentimes the impaired functioning was *because of racism.*

Like any student, I didn't know what I didn't know. I was never taught the story in its entirety. I wasn't being giving the information I needed to fully understand how ongoing discrimination in health-care settings manifests itself. As a result, I wasn't able to process all the many ways systemic racism in all aspects of society impacts health and health outcomes. And I think that has been the case for so many physicians in my generation and before me. You have this information that's withheld from you when you're a student, and as a result, you can't do your job entirely effectively or take care of people the way you should. There's a myth of objectivity that gets perpetuated, and it starts in medical school—this idea that because you're a doctor and a scientist, you're objective, you can't be biased, you can't be racist, and you don't have blind spots when it comes to your patients. But the reality is that racism absolutely exists in medicine, it's existed throughout history, and it's still hurting—and often killing—Black Americans. As our present-day medical students sit in the lecture halls and classrooms of our academic medical institutions diligently scrawling down their notes, *this* is what we need to teach them.

FIVE

Misdiagnosed

Despite the many gaps in my education at Harvard Medical School, there was one experience from my time there that became foundational to my understanding of medicine, and that was my experience as a patient. I feel extremely fortunate that I've always been healthy. I rarely get sick, and when I do, it's the usual brief cough or cold. It wasn't until I got to medical school that I had my first brush with an illness that progressed to the point where it became so serious that I almost lost my life.

I was in the middle of pharmacology class—sitting in one of those cavernous lecture halls with steep stairs and three large green chalkboards lined up at the front—when I first started feeling strange. I loved Pharm, as we referred to the first-year Pharmacology course, because we got to learn about how drugs are used to treat and manage diseases. This was a chance to apply some of the biochemistry principles we were learning to real-life scenarios. That particular day, the professor was teaching us about calcium channel blockers, which can lower blood pressure by preventing calcium from entering the cells of your heart and arteries. They really are quite powerful medications, and I was paying close attention.

As I was sitting there, my stomach began to churn, and I started feeling nauseated. I ran to the bathroom. It wasn't pretty—I had a lot of diarrhea. I went to find my sister and told her that I wasn't feeling well. Oni drove me home. On the way, I vomited all over the inside of our car. Back at the apartment, I crawled into bed. I knew something was wrong; I was having intense abdominal pain. I thought maybe I had food poisoning from a Caesar salad wrap I'd eaten the day before. Oni finally told me that she thought we should go to the emergency room.

I didn't want to go. It was one thing to study medicine, but to be a patient felt scary to me. I felt vulnerable. In fact, I hated the very idea of the hospital. Ever since our mother got sick and we'd had to spend weekends in her hospital room, I wanted to avoid them at every chance I got. Just the idea of going to the ER made me miss my mother more than ever. I was sick and frightened; I didn't know what was wrong with me. My mother had the kind of mix of firm love and tenderness that I needed at a moment like this. Instead, it was Oni who was loving and firm with me—she persuaded me to get in the car and go.

We drove over to one of the Harvard teaching hospitals. By this point, I was sick enough that I could barely stand or speak. When we arrived there, my sister had to register me. The abdominal symptoms were so bad that at one point I lay on the floor of the waiting room in the fetal position, rocking back and forth. We waited for what seemed like an eternity. Should we tell the clerk at registration at the front desk that I was a Harvard medical student? Maybe that would help me get seen faster. But I felt uncomfortable using privilege in that way, so I decided against it.

Eventually, I was called into the ER, changed into a gown, and placed on a stretcher. I was seen by multiple residents and attendings that day. The first resident was a tall young Black man I knew, as we had gone to college together. He was friendly and polite, but I could tell he felt awkward about having to care for me, given that we were acquaintances. He asked me about my symptoms, and I told him about the nausea, vomiting, diarrhea, and the intense abdominal pain.

The second was a young white woman with her brown hair up in a messy ponytail, wearing scrubs and the usual Patagonia jacket with the Harvard residency program insignia on it. She wasn't overly warm or friendly. She asked me about my symptoms, and I repeated what I had told the first resident.

She nodded and then began another line of questioning.

"Are you sexually active?" she asked.

I told her that I hadn't been sexually active in over a year and that I didn't have a partner. Although I'd had a boyfriend in Chicago, we'd broken up and were no longer together.

"I want to make sure we're considering all possible diagnoses at this point," she told me, "including sexually transmitted diseases."

She explained she wanted to do a pelvic exam to check for pelvic inflammatory disease, an infection of the reproductive organs transmitted during sex. She went ahead and did an exam, taking the speculum and opening up my cervix while pressing down hard on my abdomen. I was in enough pain already and so this exam, uncomfortable at the best of times, was excruciating, all but taking the breath out of my body.

Finally, I was seen by the attending physician. He was an older, serious-looking white man with glasses whom I recognized from clinical observation in the ER earlier in the year. What I remembered most about him from observation was that he barely acknowledged my presence, even though I was standing at his elbow. Now that I was his patient, he asked me a few questions about my pain and pushed on my tender abdomen, then said he would order some blood tests, but not any kind of imaging studies. I think he spent a grand total of about two minutes with me before he left. On his way out I heard him say to the resident that he was ruling out appendicitis because I didn't seem to be in that much pain. I never saw him again.

When the bloodwork came back, the resident came in and told me that she had talked to the attending physician and that the most likely diagnosis was gastroenteritis. She told me confidently that because I was able to keep down fluids, I could go home. I started getting dressed, and my sister, who was a year ahead of me at HMS—whispered to me, "Are they sure it's not appendicitis?" We were so early in our medical training that neither of us felt confident or empowered enough to speak up. The attending physician had made his assessment and we had to assume he knew what he was talking about. So, we left.

I spent the next day lying in bed with nausea and abdominal pain, wondering when these horrible symptoms would end. Oni was tending to me at home, but she also needed to get her studying done, and so she'd check in on me periodically, bringing me my favorite hot tea with milk and sugar to drink because I couldn't keep down any food. The next day, I was no better and so I decided to go to student health services, where I saw the nurse practitioner. I had chosen this nurse practitioner for my primary care at the beginning of the year because she had such a warm demeanor, and she seemed like she would listen to me. That day, she paid close attention to what I was telling her, examining my belly, and telling me that, like Oni, she was concerned that I had appendicitis. She sent me straight to another ER for a CT scan.

This time my ER experience was different, perhaps because I came with a note from the nurse practitioner saying a CT scan of my abdomen was indicated. At the hospital, they did the scan, but still managed to come back with a misdiagnosis of colitis—an inflammation of the colon, likely from infection.

I was put on intravenous antibiotics for a night. Thanks to the antibiotics, I felt temporarily better, but after I was discharged and sent home the next day, I was still horribly sick. The nausea had returned. The abdominal pain had worsened. I felt cold, like it was freezing, shaking and shivering all over, uncontrollably so. Later, I would come to find out that the medical term for this is *rigors*, and they happen when you are badly infected and there's bacteria in the blood. Oni took me back to the same ER. I can't even remember who was caring for me or what was said by then, I was in so much discomfort. This time, they repeated the CT scan and finally someone came in to give me the correct diagnosis.

"You have appendicitis," the resident told me gravely. "Because it wasn't caught soon enough, it ruptured. We need to operate immediately."

Everything happened so quickly, I didn't have time to ask why my inflamed appendix hadn't shown up on the prior scan. Suddenly, five or six people were around my bedside, preparing me for surgery. The new CT scan had shown my appendix was perforated, so the senior resident and the rest of the team came downstairs to the ER to make sure I was okay. They needed to get me to the OR as soon as possible. I was in danger, they told me, of losing my life.

I was terrified. I'd never gone under anesthesia or needed surgery before. I looked at Oni and she held my hand tightly, the look on her face mirroring my own fear and concern. The resident explained the procedure to me, but his words didn't fully register. The last thing I remember is someone starting the anxiolytic medicine through my IV and Oni giving me a kiss on my forehead and saying she loved me before they wheeled me into the OR, and I vanished into my dream world. When I woke up, I was in the recovery room. Hours had passed. I was groggy and my abdomen was sore. I lifted up the sheet and saw bandages over my right lower abdomen and a drain with yellow-white fluid coming out the side. I couldn't move, but I was alive.

The surgeon came in. He was a short middle-aged white man, very matter-of-fact, but clearly concerned about me. He explained he had to cut open my abdomen instead of the usual laparoscopic approach, which meant I was going to have a substantial scar and a longer recovery time. Apparently, there was so much pus in my abdomen from the rupture, there was no other way to remove the appendix and the havoc it had caused in my body.

But this wasn't the end of my troubles. I was discharged home three days later, still not feeling like myself. While much of the pain in my abdomen was gone, my belly felt large and full, and I was still nauseated. At my follow-up visit a week later with my surgeon, he examined me and told me he was worried. He sent me back to the same ER for another CT—my third—and they found that my abdomen had not been washed out thoroughly after the surgery, which can happen after a perforated appendicitis, and I had developed an intra-abdominal abscess—an accumulation of pus—that needed to be drained. I was readmitted the hospital.

I just wanted to feel better again. Why was I still sick? It was one thing after another and I had absolutely no control over anything. By now, I was already a week behind on my schoolwork; I felt confused and frustrated. I essentially had to leave my life in the hands of these physicians, but how could I trust them when it had taken them so long to give me a correct diagnosis? I felt certain that if my mother had been there at my bedside to advocate for me, the outcome might have been different. Certainly, Oni tried.

In total, I was out of school for about five weeks with postoperative complications. Most people who have appendicitis recover after a few days. A couple of months after my surgery, when I was finally regaining some normality, I happened to be walking down Longwood Avenue, the main drag in front of HMS, when I ran into the young Black surgical resident I had seen when I first came to the emergency room with my symptoms. He recognized me immediately and stopped to ask me how I was doing. I told him I was slowly getting better. The resident then explained that everyone felt horrible about what had happened, especially as I was a student at the medical school. He shared with me that because my case was a delayed diagnosis with complications, it was being presented at a morbidity and mortality conference in the Department of Surgery. They needed to review exactly what had happened and what had gone wrong. These conferences are a tradition in medicine and surgery departments. The case is presented to the whole department, the people involved in the case discuss their thoughts, and then there is an open discussion about what can be learned.

Certainly, it's not unusual for appendicitis to be misdiagnosed, so it likely wouldn't have been the first time doctors had met to discuss a failed diagnosis scenario with this problem. Overall, as many as 30 percent of patients with appendicitis are discharged by a physician before a correct diagnosis is made. Does this mean that the misdiagnosis that had cost me so many weeks of school and could have taken my life was simply an awful mistake? Many times since then, I have wondered if the color of my skin was a factor in my misdiagnosis. The second resident I saw, the white woman, was fixated on my sexual activity. Why was she so convinced I had a sexually transmitted infection despite my clear answers about *not* being sexually active? To me, this may point to some unconscious biases on her part. Negative images or stereotypes of Black women have been a pervasive part of our culture throughout American history. The idea that Black women are sexually promiscuous or lascivious or Jezebels continues to be promulgated in books, film, TV, and other cultural references to this day. It's entirely possible that this influences the ways that healthcare professionals make assumptions about Black women's sexual activity and promiscuity that, in turn, affect communication and clinical decision-making.

The very fact that the second resident didn't listen to me in that initial evaluation makes me question everything else about the way I was treated. Why did the attending doctor who saw me that first day so grossly underestimate my pain level, therefore ruling out a correct diagnosis of appendicitis? Would he have underestimated the pain of a white patient in the same way? Why did it take my nurse practitioner listening to me to reach the correct diagnosis? And why, even after she ascertained what was wrong with me, was I still given an incorrect diagnosis of colitis? The answer is: I don't know for certain. I'll never know if racism was a factor or not. This is part of the problem. It's much easier to explain blatant acts like burning crosses and racial slurs than it is to explain unconscious bias in medical settings. I don't know what was discussed at the conference about my case, just as I don't know whether bias influenced my doctors' clinical decision-making and whether someone with white skin might have ended up in the same situation. Toni Morrison once wrote, "The function, the very serious function of racism is distraction." Sometimes you just don't know if that's what's going on—and you waste hours of your life trying to figure it out.

No matter the nuances of *my* misdiagnosis, numerous case studies have shown patterns of doctors' failure to listen, failure to engage, and failure to correctly estimate the level of pain in Black patients. A 2016 report by researchers at two cancer hospitals in Michigan who looked at interactions between non-Black oncologists and their Black patients found that the oncologists with a higher level of bias spent far less time with Black patients and answered fewer questions. The meta-analysis of twenty years of studies that looked at different sources of pain in numerous settings found that Black patients were 22 percent less likely than white patients to receive pain medication when they needed it. A 2020 study indicated that Black and Hispanic children brought to emergency rooms with fractures were less likely to receive opioids for pain and were also less likely to have their pain well controlled than white children. Papers like these clearly indicate patterns that go far beyond my anecdotal evidence and point to broad systemic issues. Looking back from the vantage of the present day, it's clear to me that whether the medical professionals caring for me were motivated by bias or not, they risked my life with their misdiagnoses.

That formative experience as a patient gave me something that my professors in medical school failed to offer me: direct experience of what it feels like to be a Black patient at the mercy of the white medical establishment. Part of the reason I have the career I have today—making sure patients are listened to, that they are given care that is responsive to their needs, and that physicians aren't overlooking their pain simply because of the color of their skin—is due to that time spent as a patient, feeling vulnerable, scared, and unsure.

PART II

OPENING MY EYES

SIX

Homecoming

To this day, it still surprises me that I chose emergency medicine as my specialty. Working in an ER is an incredibly unpredictable experience, and there's this assumption that ER physicians thrive on the unexpected. That's not me: I'm someone who enjoys predictability and very much dislikes surprises. Entering medical school, I'd initially assumed I would want to specialize in hematology and oncology, having lost my mother to a blood cancer like leukemia. It was only after taking a required anatomy class during my first year at HMS that I began to consider emergency medicine instead.

My anatomy lab section was taught by a popular instructor—a charismatic, bespectacled emergency medicine physician who offered students the opportunity to shadow him in the ER at Massachusetts General Hospital, one of Harvard's teaching hospitals. I was intrigued by the opportunity and signed up right away. That night, while shadowing him, I felt myself strongly drawn to emergency medicine. As we walked from room to room seeing patients, I was in awe of my instructor's confidence and kindness. He was without fear. In a few seconds—given the lack of time you have in the ER—he would make assessments and truly connect with people.

One patient was a very tall young man who had presented to the ER with right-sided chest pain that worsened with deep breaths. My instructor introduced himself, shook hands with the young man, and then sat at eye level with him in a chair next to the bed. We had been taught in our patient-doctor course that sitting down at eye level makes patients feel more comfortable—this was something he had clearly perfected. Next, he introduced me as his student and asked the patient if I could listen to his lungs with my stethoscope. The patient said yes. As I placed the stethoscope to the man's chest, I could hear the breath sounds clearly over the left chest wall as he inhaled and exhaled, but no breath sounds on the right. The chest X-ray confirmed my instructor's suspicions. The patient had a collapsed right lung. I watched as the man underwent a bedside procedure, called a thoracostomy, to place a chest tube in order to re-expand his lung. It was nothing short of miraculous—the tube entering the layers of his chest wall, skin, subcutaneous fat, muscle, then, pop, into the chest cavity. The procedure quite simply saved his life. In that patient's room, everything I had learned in anatomy class came to life in front of my very eyes and ears.

I learned that emergency medicine is a specialty that requires a unique mix of skills. My instructor needed to think on his feet, figuring out what was required in the moment before acting thoughtfully but decisively to treat someone. This was hands-on and exciting, as you could do a huge amount to help patients, often within minutes. Conversely, he also slowed down enough to form a bond with a patient he'd never met before, earning someone's confidence at a moment of peak crisis. I noticed that if there wasn't a chair at the bedside, he would always ask the patient if it was okay if he sat at the foot of the bed. Some patients he met with that night were just scared. Some had incredibly serious conditions. Some were too ill to show any emotions at all. But no matter what the patient was going through, my instructor sat down, listened intently, examined them, and then discussed his plan.

"In emergency medicine, you get to be a generalist," he pointed out to me. "You have to know a little bit about every aspect of medicine because you see such a breadth of cases. It never gets dull."

I realized it was no coincidence that there was a long-running TV show set in an emergency room. The ER is an incredibly compelling place where you see all kinds of patients and cases, interacting with so many people in a single night. I also naively appreciated the idea of helping all comers—regardless of socioeconomic or health insurance status or demographic group. That night at Mass General, although the patient population was predominantly white, we saw several patients of color, people who had come to the ER because they had no place else to go, because they were either uninsured or didn't have access to quality care elsewhere. Like so many ERs around the country, Mass General was providing access to care at all hours of the day, where people could receive comprehensive treatment regardless of their insurance status—and whether they had a genuine health-care emergency or not.

Another patient we met with that night was a young woman from Cape Verde. She hadn't been able to make it to a doctor's appointment to get her checkup, because she was a single mother working two jobs, and her employer wouldn't give her time off work without docking her pay. She needed her blood pressure medicine refilled, and while she may not have appeared to be in need of urgent care, she knew—as we did—that if she didn't take her medicine she would be at higher risk of a stroke or a heart attack. She was seen by my instructor and left with a new prescription of lifesaving pills.

For my part, I left the hospital that night with a sense that I had found my calling.

As a student, I had yet to question the context for what was happening in the emergency room setting. Because the US lacks a single-payer, universal health-care system, access to health care in this country has long depended on insurance and a person's ability to pay, with patients of color making up a disproportionate number of the under- or uninsured. This trend dates back to the mid-twentieth century, a period when medical technology improved substantially, and visits to hospitals increased. Although insurance policies at the time covered hospital visits, they didn't tend to cover outpatient office visits, and so people without insurance found that they could access no-cost care through hospital emergency rooms instead. Emergency rooms became medical safety nets, the places where everyone could go to receive treatment regardless of their insurance status or ability to pay.

As a result, the history of emergency medicine is bound up in the experiences of Black and Latinx communities' ongoing exclusion from the health-care setting as well as our struggles for inclusion within the health-care system. Prior to the 1960s, the vast majority of hospitals in the United States were segregated by race, or they had separate wings or staff for patients strictly stratified according to skin color. Many Black communities in the South simply had no access to hospitals at all. After the passage of the Civil Rights Act in 1964, Title VI of the act mandated that any hospital that practiced racial discrimination would have federal funding withheld from it. Around the country, institutions that had systematically excluded Black patients were being forced to open their doors to everyone. Just as schools were being integrated during this period, so were hospitals.

Concurrently, a new medical specialty was emerging: emergency medicine. Until the mid-1960s, emergency rooms tended to be staffed by a motley crew of interns and residents, supervised by whatever physician happened to be on call, with specialists moonlighting on the wards when they were available. There was no such thing as physicians who were trained specifically in providing emergency care. The first ever EM training program in the country started at Cincinnati General in the late 1960s, after Black residents in the area marched on the hospital in protest against the long waiting times and subpar treatment they were receiving there. At that time, the emergency department at Cincinnati General was staffed only by trainees, patients had to wait many hours to be seen, and the quality of care was shoddy. Inevitably, medical errors were made. In response to the protests, the University of Cincinnati began its landmark emergency medicine residency training in 1970, which led to other academic medical centers across the country following suit.

The field of paramedicine also grew out of this era of civil protest. While most cities in the 1960s had private ambulance services, at the time, ambulance staff weren't trained in emergency care and they tended to service predominantly white communities. That changed in 1967 when a group of Black leaders in the Hill District of Pittsburgh approached a physician at their local Presbyterian University Hospital with an idea to provide better transportation to hospitals for their community. Up to that point, Black residents were expected to call the police when they needed transportation to a hospital. Wait times for transport could be long, with many patients understandably reluctant to call the police due to the history of police brutality and abuse against Black communities. Meanwhile, many people—Black and white— were dying on their way to hospital, deaths that could have been avoided if ambulance personnel were trained in emergency care. The physician at Presbyterian University Hospital, Dr. Peter Safar, agreed to begin training Hill District residents—many of whom had been unemployed for long periods of time—in providing emergency medical care to patients while in transit. And so, the first mobile emergency medicine program in the country was born. This all-Black paramedic service helped to establish a training model for care that was eventually implemented across the country.

Perhaps because emergency medicine grew out of the need for poor and historically underserved communities to have better access to care, there has always been a perceived commitment within the specialty to serve vulnerable populations. Emergency medicine physicians have long taken great pride in the fact that we provide care to our patients regardless of their insurance status. In 1986, this became law with the passage of the Emergency Medical Treatment and Active Labor Act, which created a federal right to emergency care for everyone. Today, nearly half of all medical treatment in the US occurs in emergency medicine departments.

I felt that I too could have a role in working in service to my community, and so when it came time to select my fourth-year clinical rotations, I chose to do my elective rotation in emergency medicine. I did three one-month electives in emergency medicine, including a rotation at Mount Auburn Hospital in Cambridge, a smaller community hospital where we saw patients from all kinds of backgrounds. Here, I could really get my feet wet. As a student in the larger teaching hospitals like Mass General, my role was more that of an observer than a clinician-to-be. At Mount Auburn, I was directly supervised by attending physicians and able to give substantial input into decisions about my patients' management plans.

My time at Mount Auburn confirmed for me that I wanted to work in the ER setting with disenfranchised populations. I wanted to be there for patients in their most vulnerable moments. It felt natural for me to take on the role of comforter and caretaker, as I noticed myself drawn to patients who seemed fearful. Due to my mom's experience being sick, I knew how unsettling and downright scary being a patient in the hospital could be. It was instinctive for me to sit with an elderly woman who was suspected of having a stroke, who was terrified to go into an MRI machine, talking her through her concerns and allaying her worries enough to help get her through the procedure. If a young boy was anxious, refusing his IV because he was too scared of the needle, I wanted to be there for him and for his mother too, comforting both of them as best I could. There was something I found deeply fulfilling about these interactions. I also enjoyed the camaraderie and the team-based environment of the ER. As an emergency medicine physician, you never work alone. You're always communicating and collaborating with all the other physicians, physician assistants, nurses, and technicians on your shift. The goal is to give rapid and competent care to each patient, efficiently evaluating their symptoms, performing a physical exam and selecting the appropriate laboratory tests or radiology exam, ruling out the most life-threatening diagnoses, and either sending them home, observing, or admitting them—and you can only do that with the support of others. An emergency department may look like a chaotic place, but it's organized chaos, with a team of people continually making thoughtful but swift decisions in the patients' best interests.

Quite simply, I loved it.

As I prepared to graduate from HMS, the time came to choose where I wanted to go for my residency. While my peers were vying for competitive residencies at prestigious, well-known institutions they saw as launching pads for highly successful careers, my heart was set on returning to Brooklyn. I knew I wanted to make a difference within my community, just as my mother had. At HMS, I had found myself mostly supervised by white residents and attending physicians, alongside my white peers—I often was the only Black person in the room. In such situations, I felt as if I were under a microscope, always hyperaware of how I spoke, the words I used, the way I dressed. I found my body would stiffen up as I walked into a patient's room. I'd stand up straight, trying to project confidence, to prove myself. I didn't know the term for what I was doing, but now I can see that it was what is known as "stereotype threat"—a psychological phenomenon in which an individual feels at risk of confirming a negative stereotype about a group they identify with. I was changing my speech, appearance, and behavior to fit in, to make others, namely white folks, feel more comfortable. If I did see another Black person working within the HMS hospitals, it was usually a member of the housekeeping or janitorial staff. We would always make eye contact, gently nod, and smile at each other. Sometimes, they would pull me aside and say they were proud of me, much like an auntie or uncle—brief exchanges that left me hungry for more of this kind of connection and warmth.

And so I chose to do my residency at Kings County Hospital/ SUNY Downstate, the same hospitals my mother had spent the bulk of her career, where I knew I would be right at home, literally and figuratively.

My medical school adviser was a kind, distinguished white endocrinologist who had been at HMS for decades.

"Are you happy, Uché?" I remember him asking me on Match Day, after I found out I had been matched with my first-choice program for emergency medicine residency.

I was overjoyed. But he had a concerned look on his face, as if somehow I were throwing away my world-class education to go back to Brooklyn. It was true that most HMS graduates wanted to train at a Harvard teaching hospital or some other elite institution, but I had seen the impact my mother had made during her career. I was going back to be closer to her, in a community that was so important to our entire family. I felt that caring for patients within my community would be much more meaningful to me than training at one of the Harvard teaching hospitals. Perhaps I could even have more of an impact.

To my knowledge, I was the first medical student at HMS ever to match at Kings County/SUNY Downstate.

I moved back to New York City—and Oni moved too. She had matched in primary care and internal medicine at Montefiore Medical Center in the Bronx and was excited about her residency program because her training curriculum was grounded in social justice. For the first time in years, we decided not to live with each other. We had studied together and earned our MD degrees together, but now it was time for a break. At our apartment in Boston, we had begun bickering over little things like who did the dishes and who took out the garbage. We were like an old married couple. Except that we weren't married, we were sisters, and we weren't children anymore. We were twenty-eight years old. Oni moved into her own place in Manhattan, and I found a home back in Brooklyn.

As a little girl, I used to love to play dress-up, wearing my mother's white lab coat. I'd rummage through her closet to find one that was freshly laundered, pulling it down from the hanger, trying it on, twirling around in front of our floor-length mirror, usually tripping over it because it was too big for me. Walking the hallways at Kings County as an adult, I felt a lot like that little girl again, wearing my new, slightly ill-fitting, oversize coat. Of course, I missed my mother, but following in her footsteps meant I was fulfilling my obligation to continue her legacy because her life had been unexpectedly cut short.

Being back at Kings County also meant encountering all kinds of familiar places daily. There was the cafeteria, where Oni and I used to do our homework after school, which still had the same red Jell-O on the menu that we used to eat all the time as kids, as well as the delicious baked chicken with mashed potatoes that had filled our tummies after school. The hospital auditorium, where I once sat, riveted, hearing my mother deliver a talk, looked the exact same way it had since the last time I was there, with its outdated wooden chairs, looking like it hadn't been renovated since the 1970s. Often, I walked by the clinic where our mother used to see her patients and where Oni and I used to sneak in to watch her.

To my relief, I found I was no longer always in the minority. At Kings County, although many of the supervising physicians were white, on some shifts, both my senior resident and attending physician would be Black. This felt quite special, especially given that Black physicians comprise such a small percentage of all physicians in the US. Many of us were from the same communities as our patients—who were mostly Black American or Afro-Caribbean—and so we talked to one another and to our patients as if we were all connected, as if we were family. I didn't have to worry about feeling outside my element; here I could be my authentic self.

Another benefit of being at Kings County was I had the privilege of working alongside people who had known and worked closely with my mother. One of her colleagues, an older Black physician from Panama, Dr. Reinaldo Austin, had worked in the ER for twenty-five years. The first time I ran into him in the hallways of Kings County, he looked at me, smiled widely, and bellowed, "Hello, Dr. Blackstock!" To hear that name from his lips, a salutation that had only been directed at my mother, floored me. I smiled back, feeling the tears well up in my eyes, as I slowly exhaled a long breath filled with both grief and pride. Dr. Austin had been extremely fond of my mother and quickly took me under his wing. After that, whenever I was on a shift with him, I knew he was looking out for me.

There were challenges ahead, for sure. I had left the extremely well-resourced Harvard institutions to work at a severely under-resourced public hospital during a period when the need for emergency services in New York City and across the country was substantial—and growing. A 2017 study out of the University of Maryland School of Medicine examined data from 1996 to 2010, finding that emergency room visits increased by 44 percent during that period, rising to 130 million in 2010. Of all the groups surveyed, Black patients were significantly more likely than other groups to visit emergency rooms because they were more likely to be uninsured and therefore more likely to use the ER to seek primary care. In 2010, patients identifying as African American used the emergency rooms 54 percent of the time, as opposed to seeing a primary care physician or health-care professional, and that number rose to 59 percent in urban areas, far higher than their white counterparts.

The patients we saw at the Kings County ER were predominantly Black and faced myriad and often complex needs. The attitude of the medical and nursing staff was one of fierce commitment: we knew we needed to do right by our patients—and we did whatever we needed to do to make that happen. But the reality was that due to our hospital's ongoing lack of funding, we were working within serious constraints. New York City has one of the largest public hospital systems in the US, with eleven acute-care hospitals serving more than a million patients each year. Patients who come to these hospitals are mostly on Medicaid or uninsured, yet despite the massive need, these hospitals continually face budget gaps. In 2006, when I came to work at Kings County, the New York City Health and Hospitals Corporation, which runs Kings County and the other ten public hospitals in the city, was facing a projected deficit of $579.2 million.

As a result of the immense need and this dire funding gap, the Kings County ER was a crowded, noisy, and often chaotic place. We never had enough nursing and ancillary staff. During my shifts, I wasn't just administering to my patients' acute health-care needs. I found myself taking care of their many other needs too: checking on prescriptions to make sure they were filled, calling family members to make sure patients had someone to pick them up, staying on hold for what seemed like forever with a specialist to ensure a patient had adequate follow-up care, contacting the social worker to make sure a patient could sign up for emergency health insurance and wasn't left with a huge bill. I would often get so backed up with patients that sometimes patients waited hours to be seen. If I left a shift at eleven p.m. and came back at three the next afternoon I might see the same patients still waiting from the night before. Or I'd return from several days off to find the same patient still waiting in the ER to be admitted to a hospital bed on the inpatient ward.

Compared with Harvard, where there were more than enough resources and staff to allow a team-based approach to caring for patients, the atmosphere in the Kings County ER was "catch as catch can," and I got all the hands-on experience I had been craving. I regularly found myself drawing blood or placing IVs because there wasn't a phlebotomist to take care of that. It wasn't unusual for me to have to mix the contrast cocktail for patients to drink before their CT scans, and I grew accustomed to transporting my patients to their imaging studies. At the beginning of my tenure at Kings County, I didn't mind having to do everything. I was getting by on excitement and adrenaline, eager to learn all I could. Every time I stepped foot in the hospital, it felt like I was encountering the full gamut of medical scenarios.

It's often said that while you get your MD in medical school, you really become a physician during residency. Residency is where you learn how to take care of your patients. Internship is the special name given to the first year of residency, a time when you finally have your own patients whom you examine, order lab tests or radiology exams and specialist consults for, and decide, based on all that information, whether to discharge home, observe in the ER, or admit to the hospital.

I remember always feeling anxious during the first days of intern year. Sometimes the night before a shift, I could barely sleep. No one expected too much from us as interns. We weren't going to be the fastest or most efficient at seeing patients, but we were expected to be thorough. The shifts were grueling. They were all twelve hours long and we usually would have four or five shifts a week, sometimes during the day from seven a.m. to seven p.m., sometimes swing shifts from eleven a.m. to eleven p.m., which were the busiest, and then the overnights, seven p.m. to seven a.m.

Often, I would forget to eat the meal that I'd packed for myself and brought in my backpack. My sandwich or snacks would remain there for the entire shift. Every now and then, I'd munch on some dried apple slices, a favorite snack of mine that my mother had introduced me to when I was a little girl. I noticed that my scrubs got much looser on me as my intern year progressed. The time between twelve-hour shifts often became a blur and consisted mostly of showering, sleeping, and working out. Once on a series of overnight shifts, there was construction with loud drilling being done on the facade of my apartment building. I had taken Benadryl to help me sleep during the day, but I was unsuccessful because of the loud noises. I got out of bed groggy, made my way to work, and realized that I was so tired that I had forgotten to put on a bra and underwear under my scrubs. I felt incredibly uncomfortable and exposed during the entire shift, utterly embarrassed, though probably no one could tell.

During another set of exhausting overnight shifts, I remember trying to collect a urine sample from an elderly patient. She had come in with fever and symptoms of a bladder infection, and I needed to send a clean urine specimen to the lab. Due to her other medical conditions, she was unable to get out of the bed on her own and I offered to place a straight urinary catheter to collect the sample. She refused. She told me she wanted to urinate on her own in the bedpan, although the cleanliness of the urine sample would be less than ideal. I gave her some fluids to drink and waited hours for her to urinate. Before she did, I cleaned her genital area myself and placed her on a bedpan. I ran to the nearest supply closet to collect the urine tubes, but by the time I returned someone had taken away the bedpan . . . and the urine sample. I stood at the bed with my arms by my sides and asked the patient, "Where did the urine go?" She replied that some lady had taken it. A well-intentioned patient care technician walked by and said, "Oh, I threw out the urine."

I replied, "Oh," as I felt my tears starting.

I ran into the hallway to finish my cry.

The patient care tech ran after me. "Oh, Dr. Blackstock, I'm so sorry. I was just trying to help."

I was in the middle of six overnight shifts in a row. I wept, slumping down onto the floor with my face in my hands.

"I'm just so tired," I sobbed.

Throughout all of this, I was aware that my problems paled in comparison to those of many of my patients. On every shift, I encountered people facing challenges that often went far beyond health issues. There was the mother who missed her follow-up appointment with a doctor for new-onset kidney failure due to her kids being home sick. She couldn't get another appointment except one that was six months away. There was the woman who had just gotten off the plane from Trinidad with a fungating breast mass that had never been treated in her own country. And the Creole-speaking elderly man who'd lost his housing, had no family, and was living in a shelter; he didn't have any diabetes medication left, as someone had stolen his last few pills at the shelter. I remember the looks on their faces, the eagerness to be helped, the appreciation that someone was taking the time to care and to listen.

Then there were the young people—Black boys, mainly—who had gotten caught up in or unwittingly caught in the middle of gang violence. The slight and lanky twelve-year-old who was walking his dog on his block in the late afternoon after school when he was caught in the crossfire between two gangs. Somehow the bullet went through his neck mere millimeters from his major neck vessels—the carotid artery and the internal jugular vein; if the bullet had hit either, he would have bled out right there in the street within seconds. Fortunately, it missed these critically important blood vessels. We were able to stabilize him and he was admitted to the hospital for a flesh wound and observation. Not all patients were so lucky. The sixteen-year-old who came in unconscious and bleeding from the back of the head, the pink tissue extruding from his scalp at the site where a bullet had entered, whose stat CT scan showed a catastrophic brain injury from the bullet. As we tried to stabilize him, we could hear someone who was likely his mother wailing outside in the hallway. I will never get over the sound of a family member crying out in grief; it is one of the most painful sounds one could ever hear. The patient had a cardiac arrest in the ER and died that same day.

Cases like these had a huge impact on all of us working in the ER. Even though, superficially, gun violence may seem to be about interactions between individuals, we were well aware of the part that social and structural issues played in cases like these. As physicians, we could patch up our patients' wounds, but for us to truly make a difference, these issues needed to be treated at their root. The trauma of poverty as well as the lack of affordable housing, quality education, and employment opportunities were major factors. My mother's friend Dr. Austin had founded Doctors Against Murder (DAM) after caring for a large number of young Black patients in the ER due to gun violence and other violent interactions. Another one of my colleagues, Dr. Rob Gore, my friend and also an attending physician, started an anti-violence program called KAVI (Kings Against Violence Initiative) because of all the Black boys and young Black men who became his patients. Their work was inspiring—it was obvious to them that to end gun violence they had to address the underlying systemic issues that often led to it; if they didn't, that violence would keep sending young men in the prime of their lives through their ER doors.

In the same way, I came to see that the woman who couldn't take time off work to get her blood pressure medication wasn't only suffering from high blood pressure, she was suffering from lack of workplace protections. The young man who lost his life to gun violence clearly needed better educational and employment opportunities. The elderly gentleman who had his diabetes medication stolen at the homeless shelter would need safe, permanent housing before his health could ever begin to improve in meaningful ways. To have people use the ER as their primary source of care spoke volumes to me about the many ways our dysfunctional and chronically underfunded health-care system was failing to meet the needs of our communities. If our government had invested the resources into robust and accessible social services, public health, primary prevention, and single-payer, universal health care in this country, many of our patients wouldn't need to be in the ER in the first place.

I had gone into the field seeing the ER as a place where I could have the opportunity to serve those most in need. As time went on, however, I came to view it as the place where the United States' social problems come home to roost.

SEVEN

Three Patients

Working in an emergency department, you rarely know your patients very well, as some will come in once, or a few times, but then you might never see them again. That wasn't the case for a patient I'll call Jordan, a thin, lanky young man suffering from sickle cell anemia. Jordan came to the ER often, usually during a sickle cell pain crisis. I'd find him lying sprawled out on a stretcher, grimacing. Although he was in his thirties, Jordan had the look of a teenager, always wearing his New York Knicks baseball cap, jean jacket, and what I had determined was his favorite pair of baggy jeans, which made him look even younger. His caramel skin was flawlessly smooth. No wrinkles, perhaps a side effect of his disease, which made his situation even more poignant, given that most people with sickle cell anemia don't live past their fortieth birthday.

According to the biomedical textbook definition, the cause of Jordan's suffering was misshapen red blood cells, which essentially get stuck in the blood vessels, resulting in less oxygen delivery throughout the body. This can lead not only to extreme pain but also to pneumonia, splenic infarctions, and even premature death. Sickle cell is an incurable and inherited disease—and it tends to be found in people with ancestors from sub-Saharan Africa; South America, the Caribbean, and Central America; Saudi Arabia; India; and Mediterranean countries such as Turkey, Greece, and Italy. However, because people from sub-Saharan Africa are racialized as Black in the US, sickle cell anemia gets inaccurately labeled as a Black disease. Today, there are one hundred thousand people in the US who have sickle cell disease, and most of them are Black. At the Harvard teaching hospitals, I had seen only a handful of patients with this disease, but there were weeks at Kings County when I felt as if I saw at least one patient suffering with sickle cell during most of my shifts. These patients would arrive at the ER often crying out for pain medication, barely able to walk or talk, clutching whichever part of them was hurting, usually an arm, leg, or their chest. Their brown skin often looked dull, which is what happens when your hemoglobin drops.

Jordan quickly became a part of my life as a resident, he was at the ER so often. When he came in, I knew that if we didn't immediately treat him with pain medication, oxygen, and fluids, then the consequences could be dire and even fatal. Most of his crises involved pain in both his legs and would usually be precipitated by a change in weather, dehydration, or even a stressful interaction. In time, I was able to quickly identify when Jordan was especially sick, and I knew which combination of pain medications worked best for him. Even if he wasn't my patient that shift, I would drop by his stretcher to say hello and to see how he was doing. He was always polite and soft-spoken. Although I didn't follow basketball, I usually asked him about his favorite team, the New York Knicks, and we'd chat for a while.

Tragically, because sickle cell disease is perceived as affecting a primarily Black population, patients like Jordan aren't always treated with the dignity and respect they deserve. At Kings County, I was saddened to find out that a few of my senior residents, some of whom had supervised me closely and whose clinical acumen I admired, held a particular attitude toward patients with sickle cell disease. Occasionally, as an intern, I would hear them speaking disparagingly about the "frequent flyers," patients who came often to the ER complaining of pain, sometimes every week, or sometimes every day for a week. The senior residents would say, "Oh that's so-and-so. Give two rounds of pain medication and then let them go." The insinuation was that the patient was drug-seeking and didn't require admission.

As a student, I recalled my deep unease in class when our white professor insisted that we needed to make sure that patients who claimed to have sickle cell were actually in pain and not drug-seeking before treating them. The implication was that we were going to see patients coming into the ER who were just trying to get high from the pain medication and weren't truly suffering from this terrible disease. We were being taught that these particular patients were not to be trusted. Would we be making the same assumption if it were a disease that affected a predominantly white population? Most likely not.

According to some of my senior residents, the best way to

determine if someone was truly in pain was by looking at their vital signs. Was the patient's heart rate fast or blood pressure high? That would clue you in to the truth, supposedly. But sometimes patients' vital signs were within normal range and they were still in obvious pain! A few of our supervising physicians even required us to run hemoglobin tests to confirm that patients had sickle cell disease and not sickle cell trait (a milder version in which people did not have pain crises). One of the old-school hematologists had come up with a pain medicine protocol for treating these pain crises, the idea being that a standardized protocol would remove the bias from clinicians. I was doing my best to listen and learn from my superiors, but at the same time I felt that having a standardized protocol could result in a patient's pain not being adequately treated. It felt counter-scientific, as pain is subjective.

When I was an intern and less experienced, I did as I was told, diligently giving patients two shots of morphine (into their deltoid muscle because we were taught giving intravenously would produce a high) before discharging them. If they needed more than two rounds of pain medication, they would have to be admitted to the hospital. I was still new to the job; I didn't want to ruffle any feathers. But as I grew more confident in my clinical skills, I began to challenge certain supervising physicians. Sometimes, I would push for a patient with sickle cell disease to be admitted to the hospital or for us to give a slightly higher dose of pain medication. I wasn't always successful, but at least I was trying to advocate for my patients.

One winter in my second year of residency, after coming back from a short vacation, I learned from my coresidents that Jordan had died. He was thirty-four. He had come into the ER a few days prior with fever, trouble breathing, and chest pain. He was diagnosed with pneumonia on chest X-ray, and admitted to the hospital for acute chest syndrome, a severe complication of sickle cell disease. Jordan ended up being admitted to the ICU for monitoring, and IV antibiotics and a breathing tube had been placed to help him breathe better. But he didn't make it. When I found out, I quickly excused myself from my duties and walked to the nearest bathroom. There, I closed the door of the stall and slumped down against it, tears pouring down my face.

In the aftermath of Jordan's death, I spent a lot of time reflecting on what I'd learned being one of his clinicians. Taking care of Jordan had taught me to always advocate for my patients despite formal medical school and residency curricula that instructed me to do otherwise. He led me to more deeply interrogate and challenge the medical system that had failed him. A few of my medical school professors and senior residents weren't the only ones suspicious of patients with sickle cell disease. In one recent study, 63 percent of nurses surveyed held the belief that many patients with the disease are addicted to opioids. In another study, led by an emergency nurse at Duke University, nurses and physicians from the emergency departments with the highest number of patients with SCD scored only a 65 out of 100 on a test assessing their knowledge of sickle cell disease. In another study, researchers found that patients with sickle cell disease wait 25 percent longer to see a doctor in the ED than do other patients, even though people with the disease tend to have worse pain.

I learned that our health-care system has never devoted enough effort and resources to finding treatments and cures for this "Black" disease. Sickle cell anemia was first identified over one hundred years ago, yet the medical establishment is still insufficiently invested in the research, care, and treatment of people with this condition. Why? Because it's perceived as affecting a predominantly Black population. When you compare the amount of research and funds given to other, similar diseases, the inequity is glaring. Hemophilia, another inherited disease, affects around 20,000 mostly white people a year. There are 28 drugs to treat hemophilia. Meanwhile, sickle cell disease affects a much larger population—100,000 mostly Black people per year—but it has only two FDA-approved drugs for treatment. Cystic fibrosis affects 30,000 mostly white people, one-third the number of people with sickle cell disease, but receives three to four times more federal research funding per person.

Despite the lack of overall investment in ameliorating suffering from sickle cell disease, there are those who have long advocated for sickle cell patients. In the early 1970s, the Black Panthers recognized how much this particular disease had been neglected by the establishment and so they began conducting community outreach, organizing a national screening program using rapid testing and even working with medical students to visit people in their homes and administer screening tests. Today, there are passionate and dedicated researchers who work on identifying better treatments and even a cure—but they need far more support and funding than they currently receive. As long as the medical community at large accepts the preposterous idea that the biology of

Black patients is inferior to that of white patients, and until we upend the idea that the problem with sickle cell disease lies with Black people themselves, rather than with fallacious perceptions and inequities in treatment, patients like Jordan will continue to suffer and even die.

The day that I found out about Jordan's death was one of many moments that radicalized me as a physician. My professors at HMS and my senior residents would have doubtlessly applied a biomedical perspective on Jordan's early death, convinced that his "abnormal" red cells due to an inherited condition were to blame, that it was "just bad luck" that he was born with them. I came to understand that a more accurate interpretation was that Jordan and patients like him were at the mercy of a health-care system that did not always view them as deserving of high-quality, compassionate, and sometimes lifesaving care. Once I began to see the failures of our health-care system to take care of Black people, I couldn't stop seeing them.

There were examples everywhere.

Unlike my experience with Jordan, I met with the young pregnant woman only once. I will never forget her. It was very late at night and I had to call out for her a few times before finally locating her in a corner of the waiting area, curled up on a stretcher under a mound of white hospital sheets. This often would happen at the ER, that I would have to walk around the waiting area multiple times to find a patient. If this had been a better-resourced hospital, the ER would have been less crowded, more orderly, with assigned rooms and enough nurses and ancillary staff. I wouldn't have had to go searching for a patient in order to treat her.

The young woman emerged from under the sheets. I could see she was petite, with smooth brown skin. She was wearing a thin, flimsy hospital gown, and a scarf on her head covered her hair. It was clear she was in pain—her face was creased in a frown and both her arms were wrapped around her abdomen. I bent down, took her hand.

"I don't feel good, I think I'm miscarrying. Again," she said.

The young woman was only in her twenties and yet she had just told me this wasn't the first time she had gone into labor well before her due date.

I knew that I needed to examine her and would have to perform an emergency pelvic ultrasound. For this, I needed a private exam room, but these were rarely available at Kings County because we had only four of them in the ER. I quickly rounded the hallways and was relieved when I found an empty room, even if it was still messy from the last patient encounter. I rushed to tidy it up, getting all my supplies together, including a speculum for a pelvic exam and lots of absorbent pads to place under her. Then I went back to find my patient, and rolled her on her stretcher over to the exam room, helping her up onto the table, using one of the sheets from her stretcher to place across her lap. I asked her to lean back as I put down the back of the exam table, and then I pulled out the stirrups for her to put her feet into, so that I could perform a thorough pelvic exam. I put on my gloves. I began saying the words I'd say to any patient during one of these exams:

"This is my hand as I rest it on your inner thigh. You're going to feel some pressure. I'm going to use my gloved fingers to help me to place the speculum in your vagina...."

And as I placed the speculum, that's when it happened. The tiny fetus slipped out into my hands. I stared down at the tiny creature, shocked because it was still moving ever so slightly, its skin translucent. It was probably about fourteen weeks old. Nothing I'd learned in medical school had prepared me for this moment, but I told myself to stay present for my patient. I quickly regained my composure and explained to the young woman on the table what had happened, that she had miscarried and passed the fetus. She had been straining her head up to listen to me. Now she dropped it back on the backrest as if defeated. I thought carefully about what to do next. I decided if it were me, I would want to hold my baby and so I asked my patient if she would like that too.

"Yes," she told me, her voice a whispered rasp.

So I wrapped the tiny fetus in one of the absorbent pads and put the bundle gently in her arms.

My patient began crying softly as she held her baby. I told her that I would give her some time to be alone. I left her in the room for about fifteen minutes, took a walk around the ER to check on my other active patients. When I returned, she was still cradling her bundle, rocking it gently in her arms. I told her that I would have to send the fetus to pathology to be studied. With infinite care and love, she placed it in the small container I offered and then turned her face away into the exam table, sobbing. I knew this young woman had arrived at the ER alone, so I called the OB-GYN consult resident to come see her to ensure that she had follow-up. I wished I could have hugged her, but the interactions in the ER are always so fleeting.

After I left my shift that night, I couldn't stop thinking about this young woman—wondering if everything had been done that could be done. Most EM physicians don't stop thinking about our patients when we leave the hospital. We ruminate about them while lying in bed trying to fall asleep at night and while standing in the shower stall listening to the white noise of the water falling from the showerhead. We constantly ask ourselves: "Did that patient get everything they needed?" When you're multitasking, there are so many areas, so many opportunities for something to get missed, something to get dropped, that it adds another level of stress to an already stressful environment. This young woman had likely waited hours before being identified as very sick. Although it's possible she would have miscarried anyway, I couldn't help but feel that if she had received treatment sooner, perhaps the outcome would have been different.

Then I thought about all the steps or interventions that should have happened to prevent my patient from ending up in the ER in the first place, but that hadn't happened because this country has not prioritized allocating funds and resources for public health—more specifically, for primary prevention. I thought about the lack of prenatal care and support she likely experienced before coming to the ER, which may have also contributed to the miscarriage. Studies show that Black women experience pregnancy loss—whether due to miscarriage, stillbirth, or preterm birth—at much higher rates than white women. A 2013 study found that Black women experienced miscarriage more often than white women, and between the tenth and twentieth gestational weeks, Black women's rate of miscarriage was nearly twice that of white women. Even when factors such as alcohol use and age were controlled for, including early-pregnancy ultrasounds, there were no differences in the health of the pregnancy between Black and white women. This study suggests the difference in miscarriage risk may somehow be linked solely to race, and more specifically to racism. As a group, Black women in the US are less likely to have access to high-quality prenatal care, they're less likely to have health insurance, and less likely to receive adequate health care, education, and support than their white counterparts, all of which can affect pregnancy outcomes. While socioeconomic factors are important in the discussion of pregnancy loss in Black women, several studies have found that the risk exists, though to a lesser degree, even among affluent, educated Black women. Previous studies have also shown that there are differences in the quality of care delivered to Black and white patients. Black patients are monitored less closely in clinics and hospitals, which may explain the inequities in pregnancy loss.

There was probably little I could have done at that moment to prevent my patient from miscarrying. The least I could have done, which I hope I did, was to honor her humanity by showing her compassion, providing her competent care, but that wasn't enough. It was during residency that I realized it didn't matter how well intentioned I was, how good a job I wanted to do. If the system couldn't support me or others who were invested in our communities to do the work, then my patients weren't going to have the same outcomes as white patients at a well-funded hospital twenty minutes away in Manhattan.

———

My time at Kings County marked the beginning of my reeducation as a physician. As I was growing up, my parents had spoken candidly to my sister and me about racism, especially the kind they faced every day in their careers. They both regularly experienced what's known as interpersonal racism, when white people display outwardly discriminatory behavior toward Black people and other people of color. Systemic racism tends to be more insidious, and while its impact has arguably done more damage to our communities than interpersonal racism, it wasn't really a regular topic of discussion for our family at the dinner table, even if our parents must have sensed and to some degree understood the burden it placed on their lives. Maybe they were even trying to protect us, as parents sometimes do, from the depth of the problem. Arriving as a young MD in training, I was still very green. Over time, that changed—I changed. Every day in our Brooklyn ER, I witnessed how a lack of investment in health, in adequate housing, employment, and education, and the stress and trauma of racism brought people to our doors for reasons that went far beyond their biology. My colleagues were speaking to me about these issues, about cases that didn't only speak to medical needs, but that revealed the myriad ways that the structural violence of racism affects Black people's lives. I began to see all the many ways that Black communities had been served poorly, not only by the health-care system, but by a society that has always treated us as less than.

At the same time, I was waking up to all the ways in which lack of resources and a supportive infrastructure contribute to our ability to nurture our patients as physicians. Kings County had a lot of dedicated and talented staff doing everything they could to take care of our patient population. But there's only so much you can do with the tools you've been given. When I first started my residency, I thought I would want to stay at this hospital forever. I considered it my home. I wanted to work with my community, and I felt magnetically drawn to a specialty I considered my vocation. I had a feeling of connection to my patients—who reminded me of my neighbors and family members—and of course to my mother, who had worked there too. What's more, I began to gain confidence in myself at Kings County. My third year there, I decided to run for chief resident of my residency class. I was feeling the stirrings of leadership within me. There were four of us and I was the only Black person running for chief resident. All the residents and faculty in the program voted for the chief residents, so when three of my coresidents and I won (and found out that I had received the highest numbers of votes), I felt deeply proud that people had faith in me and that I had faith in myself to take a chance and run.

As I progressed through residency, my clinical responsibilities grew from managing my own patients as an intern to a supervisory role as a senior resident. As senior residents, we were responsible for "running the room." We had to keep track of all the patients in our section of the ER, know which intern or junior residents were assigned to them, know the status of the patients they were evaluating, and sometimes even manage our own patients to help out with the patient volume. Rotating medical students would present patient cases to us, and we discussed them with our attending physicians. It was often grueling work, but those final two years of residency helped to prepare us to practice independently. We knew more details about the patients in the ER than our own attending physicians did.

But as time went on, I realized I was burning out fast. As senior residents, we did a mix of mostly eight-hour shifts and then twelve-hour shifts on the weekend. We often didn't take real breaks, inhaling our lunch or dinner in minutes in front of our computers as we typed up our patient notes. Sometimes I didn't have time to use the bathroom during a shift because there was too much to do. I never, ever called out sick from work during my residency. No matter how exhausted or depleted I felt, I always dragged myself to work because I knew that we were short-staffed at the best of times. The overnights were the toughest—although it wasn't quite as busy, you were exhausted, everything just seemed to take longer to get done, and the shifts seemed to last forever. As my mother's daughter, I did everything I could to take care of my health. I went to the gym regularly and for daily runs, the rhythmic pounding of my sneakers on the sidewalks of my Brooklyn neighborhood helped to quell the frustration I was experiencing every day at work. But in the end, all the self-care in the world couldn't make up for the long hours and intense stress of the job. I began to question whether working under such conditions year after year was going to be sustainable for me—whether I should stay at Kings County after I completed residency.

I was in my fourth and final year of residency when I reached my breaking point. By then, I was a seasoned senior resident, no

longer the eager, impressionable intern I had been when I'd arrived. That day, I was taking care of an older Caribbean woman
who had come into the ER with her grandson. She had vomited
while grocery shopping with him, and he had brought her straight
to the ER. She explained that she had recently undergone abdominal surgery and had been experiencing several days of nausea
and abdominal pain. I was most concerned about a bowel obstruc-
tion related to the surgery and felt she needed a CT scan to ac-
curately diagnose her. I'd put in the order for the scan, but as was
typical, it was taking a long time. At Kings County, there was only
one CT scan machine for the entire ER and not enough technicians, so if one of the technicians went on a break, we would get
even more backed up. Clearly, one of the technicians had gone for
lunch, because although I had put the order in, it was as if it had
disappeared into a black hole. I'd been calling and calling the CT
scan room, but no one was picking up. I knew from past experience that if I wanted to get my patient her scan, I had to be asser-
tive. I had to keep pestering and pestering the CT scan team, but
in the meantime, I had dozens of other patients waiting for me. I
could feel my blood pressure rising by the minute.

My patient was in her seventies and was the kind of older
woman who usually warmed my heart, reminding me of my great-
aunt in Jamaica, a former schoolteacher, who had softened a little
in her older years but still had a fire in her. I could tell that, like my
great-aunt, my patient wasn't going to take no for an answer.

"My dear, when am I going to get my scan?" she pressed me as
I passed her stretcher in the crowded ER hallway, tugging at the
sleeve of my white coat.

"Soon," I promised her. "It might just take a bit longer because we're backed up right now."

But the CT scan didn't happen soon. Minutes turned into hours. Every time I passed her, she asked me again about her scan, advocating for herself in a way that I should have considered admirable, but that grated on my last nerve. When she asked for the fourth or fifth time, I'm embarrassed to say I snapped: "I don't know when you're going to get your scan. I would do it myself if I could, but I can't...."

To this day, I can see the look on her face as the words that I would always regret came flying out my mouth. She flinched away from me, casting her eyes downward toward the hospital floor. It was as if I had betrayed her. I hadn't yelled, but I had let my irritation and frustration show. I had disrespected her, and that was wrong. Once I cooled down, I went back and apologized to her and she was gracious enough to accept the apology.

But the fact that I didn't speak to her kindly when she had asked a very reasonable question made me realize that there was something wrong with my place of work too. After I came home that evening, I remember thinking to myself, "Uché, it's time to move on."

I wasn't alone in reaching the point of burnout. A lot of people at Kings County felt just as passionate as I did about providing health care to our patients; even so, some chose not to continue to practice medicine in this challenging environment and, reluctantly, decided to leave. Since the 2010s, the problem of clinician retention has only gotten worse, exacerbated by the COVID-19 pandemic. In July 2021, the United States Department of Health and Human Services announced that $103 million in funding for the American Rescue Plan would be allocated to address burnout in the health-care workforce. Since the start of the pandemic, it's estimated that one in five US health-care workers have quit their jobs, adding to concerns about burnout and its impact on our health-care system and, ultimately, our patients. The tragedy is that we know that Black patients have better health outcomes when they're cared for by physicians who look like them. They receive more information, communication is better, and they are more likely to follow treatment instructions. And so when even a few Black health-care professionals are not provided with enough resources or systemic support—and they end up having to leave—the loss to patients is enormous.

As my residency at Kings County was coming to an end, I decided I needed to take a mental health break before I started in a faculty position, to get my bearings together, as my mother used to say. Most people who graduate from an emergency medicine residency go into community practice, and only a small percentage apply for and are accepted into fellowships, which are extra training in a subspecialty of emergency medicine. I knew it would be helpful to have a niche if I wanted to stay in academic medicine, and so I decided to go the fellowship route, applying to a yearlong emergency ultrasound fellowship at St. Luke's Roosevelt Hospital, a private hospital system in Manhattan. Most people think of ultrasound being used to see how a pregnancy is progressing, but in the ER it's used to evaluate trauma patients for blood in the abdomen or chest, or around the heart. We can also use it to diagnose stones in the gallbladder or blood clots in the legs. I'm a visual learner, which made me love ultrasound even more, and I felt it was an important clinical diagnostic tool that helped me better care for my patients. This would be my first year as an attending physician, which meant I was going to take on a supervisory role, working part-time clinically, while using my nonclinical time to refine my emergency ultrasound skills and expertise.

To this day, I still have a tremendous amount of guilt about leaving Kings County. My mother worked in historically under-resourced hospitals throughout her career. She viewed becoming a physician as an opportunity to do important work in service to our communities, as well as a chance to have a better life for herself and her family. Even though she knew the system was essentially broken, and there were multiple barriers to our advancement, she had hoped the journey would be easier for Oni and me. But it was the opposite. Our mother had stayed at Kings County for ten years; I barely managed four. She was tougher than I was. Yet I knew that she had cared just as deeply as I did. How many times during her career had she experienced the rage and grief that came from looking after patients whose obstacles to health often seemed insurmountable? How many times had she excused herself to go to the bathroom so she could cry? And how had she had the endurance and wherewithal to work for close to two decades within systems and a society that refused to see Black people as fully human?

EIGHT

A Tale of Two Emergency Rooms

As my yearlong fellowship at St. Luke's came to an end, I decided not to go back to Kings County. Instead, I applied for a permanent faculty position at New York University School of Medicine. I saw an opportunity for myself there. The name alone carries a huge amount of gravitas, and its department of emergency medicine was particularly revered. This was a place where I could work with some of the legends in the field of emergency medicine, take advantage of a well-resourced institution, and—as my department didn't yet have a fellowship in emergency ultrasound (which was my new subspecialty)—I could develop a fellowship program there from the ground up. At the same time, I would have the chance to work at the Bellevue ER, a public hospital affiliated with NYU, which served an extremely diverse patient population. When NYU offered me the role of clinical instructor, I gladly accepted.

By now, I had also started seriously dating someone. Chris and

I had first met as kids because my father and his mother were friends. We had gone to each other's birthday parties when we were little, but we didn't reconnect until we crossed paths at various social events while I was in fellowship. What I loved most about being with Chris was how our relationship left me more balanced. I was used to focusing mostly on my work, and now I was creating room for someone else. I was also experiencing the pressure of societal expectations. In my thirties, I was getting the typical message that it was time to settle down, to start thinking about a family. I was someone who had always dutifully followed the predictable steps involved in medical training—being premed in college, going to medical school, then completing residency training, and finally fellowship. Getting a job in academic medicine while entering a committed relationship and thinking about starting a family was the natural next step for me.

Oni was also moving on. After residency, she had undertaken a one-year HIV clinical fellowship at Harlem Hospital, where our mother had trained. Here, she got to work with older physicians who had known our mother, just as I had at Kings County. After the Harlem fellowship, she completed a research fellowship program at Yale with a master's degree in health services research. Her focus was on developing interventions and programs to connect Black and Latina women to HIV care and to help support them in taking their HIV treatment. Black women are disproportionately infected with HIV, a fact that is little known to the general public. After Yale, Oni had returned to New York to become an assistant professor in the Division of General Internal Medicine at Montefiore Hospital, where she had completed her residency. She returned to Monte, as the institution is affectionately called, in part because she had a Black woman mentor there who she knew would support her as she launched her career as an academic researcher. She had gotten married, and was beginning to think about starting a family. We were both determined to walk the path our mother had laid for us, to make her proud.

—————

My first day of my new job at NYU, fresh out of fellowship, finally starting my career as faculty at a prestigious academic medical center, should have been a peak moment for me. Yet I couldn't help but worry about how I would fit in. I was hired in 2009. After asking around, I had discovered that I was the very first Black woman faculty member in my department. "Really?" I remember thinking, feeling shocked and disappointed that this kind of history was still being made. As one of the very few Black faculty members in my department, I knew there was every chance I might feel isolated or be unable to thrive, that my path might be blocked when it should have been wide open, but I tried to put such negative thoughts aside.

Walking into the main hospital building at NYU my first day, on my way to orientation, I had to pass through what's known as the Hall of Portraits. This is the long bank of paintings in gilded frames hanging in a corridor off the main lobby at Tisch Hospital. As I cast my eyes across the paintings, I registered immediately that every single one of the faces I saw in those portraits was that of a white man. Some wore glasses, some posed with microscopes, others held a pen in hand. Doubtless, these men in the pictures were physicians and surgeons who had made important scientific advancements in their respective fields over the past few centuries. Some of the paintings looked old enough that I wondered how many of their subjects had participated in and profited from slavery or had experimented on enslaved people. They certainly would have benefited from racist and sexist admission policies that had excluded people who looked like me from medicine for centuries.

As a student at HMS, I had often hurried down hallways decorated with portraits like these, too busy with my schoolwork to dwell much on the significance of these white faces in gold frames, not wanting to stop and contemplate what such images were saying to students like me about who is and isn't valued within our medical institutions. That first day at NYU, however, I chose to keep my head high. Perhaps naively, I walked past the bank of portraits with a sense that my very presence was a rebuke to the white men in those paintings, that I did belong there. Just like my white colleagues, I deserved to take my place in an institution where I could build my career and take advantage of abundant opportunities and resources. I reminded myself that it was important for me to be in these kinds of spaces so that Black students and residents could see someone who looked like them, came from the same communities as them, and cared deeply about our communities, who could mentor, motivate, and inspire them. I refused to take those portraits at face value or for what they truly were—a clear declaration of my new employer's foundational values and a celebration of a status quo that the institution was determined to enshrine.

My days as faculty were divided up between my clinical shifts in the emergency department, supervising medical students and residents, and my academic work. On the academic side, I was giving lectures to students, running workshops with residents, and engaging in educational research in ultrasound, focusing on how this technology could be better leveraged as a tool to teach anatomy and physiology. Ultrasound was an easy-to-use and convenient tool that enabled students to literally see the heart beating inside a patient's chest or the pathologic fluid floating inside the abdomen of a patient. I derived a huge amount of satisfaction from watching the light bulb go off for my students as they made the connection between what they'd learned in the classroom and what they were now seeing in their patients, right in front of them.

The other three or four days of the week, I was a practicing physician at one of two ERs. The first was at NYU Tisch, the private hospital that was part of the university. The other was at Bellevue, the public hospital affiliated with the medical school. These two ERs sit right next door to each other. Although I'd always been aware of inequities in emergency care in New York City, working in these spaces, I came face-to-face with the glaring disparities between public and private health care in my city.

The private emergency room at Tisch was nothing less than a well-oiled machine. Named for the family of billionaires who endowed the institution, Tisch Hospital was highly resourced in every way. No patient had to share a room with anyone else, every patient was accounted for, and arranging follow-up appointments was a breeze. When I put in my CT scan order, the order would magically get fulfilled—every time. Although we were dealing with a much smaller volume of patients than I had seen at Kings County, we had many more nurses per team and were much better staffed in terms of attending and resident physicians. As a result, I was able to care for many more patients on a given shift because I wasn't caught up doing extraneous tasks. There was even a more robust and user-friendly electronic medical record system.

But perhaps the biggest difference from Kings County was in the patient population. The people in the waiting room at Tisch were relatively wealthy, insured, with access to high-quality care outside the ER—and by extension, they were mostly white. Often, patients came to the Tisch ER because NYU specialists had referred them for an emergent issue. Even before they arrived at the ER, they were fully plugged into a medical system that they understood how to navigate and that understood them. These patients received rapid, individualized treatment, and immediate follow-up plans were made. Sometimes, we would get calls warning us that a "VIP" was on their way over. These VIPs were usually benefactors, board of trustees members, or even members of the Tisch family. When this happened, we'd receive multiple phone calls on our work cell phones and had to follow detailed instructions as to how to care for this patient when they arrived. Either the VIP was quickly admitted to the hospital or follow-up care was rapidly arranged.

But Tisch was only half of my clinical practice. My other shifts were spent at the Bellevue ER, part of the largest hospital in New York City and the oldest public hospital in the country. To say we saw a more diverse patient population at Bellevue would be an understatement. At Bellevue, patients came from every corner of the city—and the world. This was an ER with a reputation for being a place where no one would be turned away, regardless of their immigration status or ability to pay. In 2010, the year I arrived at NYU, the Affordable Care Act was passed, which created new health coverage options, with many uninsured becoming eligible for coverage when their states adopted Medicaid expansion under the ACA. This was excellent news and went some way toward addressing health insurance coverage inequities in our country. But at Bellevue, it didn't seem to make any dent in the numbers of people we saw on a daily basis, most of whom lacked insurance.

Like the ER at Kings County, Bellevue was a chaotic place where there were always too many patients and not enough physicians and nurses. Everything took a long time at Bellevue: the test results, the medications, the scans, all of it. I never knew what a shift would bring, and no two shifts were ever the same. The Bellevue ER sits right next door to a large men's shelter for people who are unhoused, which meant we were taking care of people struggling with lack of safe and adequate housing and a host of physical and mental health problems, including substance use disorder. The hospital was also a level 1 trauma center, so we managed many of the city's gunshot and stabbing victims, and we had a contract with the city's Department of Corrections, so people who had just been arrested came to the ER to be medically cleared before being taken to jail. I had nights on the job when I was cussed out by intoxicated patients, and when patients lashed out at me not just verbally but also physically.

I recall once going to tell a patient that I needed to arrange for him to have a blood draw. He was lying on a stretcher, under a white hospital sheet. When he didn't respond, I said his name again, this time tapping him on the shoulder, explaining why I needed his attention. Suddenly, the white sheet rose up with the man under it. He roared at the top of his lungs, spinning his body over, giving me just enough time to step out of the way as he flung the contents of a small urinal filled with his sample in my direction. The yellow liquid hit the wall behind me and dripped to the floor. I remember my feeling of relief when I looked down at my scrubs and realized that thanks to my quick response, I didn't have a single drop of his urine on me.

On any given shift, we were seeing people who had slipped through the cracks of a system that was simply not built to serve them. I can still remember the pain-stricken features of a young Black man who came in with a broken leg that had become dangerously infected. He had been hit by a car several weeks back and had been taken to one of the other ERs in the city, where he was diagnosed with a tibia-fibula fracture in his leg. He had been discharged with a splint, but because the hospital staff there hadn't arranged for proper follow-up for him, he had been sitting at home suffering in increasingly unbearable pain. Eventually, he came to us, where we diagnosed him with necrotizing fasciitis, an infection of the tissues beneath the skin, a very serious and potentially life-threatening condition that could have been avoided if he'd only been able to see a doctor many weeks ago. We would often care for patients like this who had been "lost to follow-up," which meant that although they had been treated at the time of their emergency, they hadn't been able to access care beyond that point. We would say "lost to follow-up" with an exasperated sigh, as if it was just the way things were. But it didn't explain why our medical system was so broken that people routinely did not receive the timely care they needed.

Often, I was dealing with patients battling substance use disorders; many were suffering with mental illnesses. I knew at the start of a shift that there was a chance I was going to be called the N- or the B-word. One time I was on shift with my senior resident, a young Black woman. She told me that she had just come from seeing a psychotic patient, a white woman, who was yelling the N-word repeatedly at the top of her lungs.

"The patient says she doesn't want me to see her," the resident explained, visibly shaken.

I told her I'd go and see the patient myself. As I walked into the room, the patient started screaming the same epithet, demanding that I leave the exam room. She was disheveled, her hair was a mess, her clothing stained as she paced around her stretcher. She was clearly in a bad state mentally, but as I didn't sense she was a danger to me, I went over and tried to engage her in a conversation to see if I could get her to cooperate with us. Perhaps I should have been upset at being called the N-word, but instead, I stayed calm. I knew that the number of patients needing psychiatric treatment in the city was far greater than the number of inpatient psychiatric beds available, which is why so many people like this woman ended up on the streets and in the city's emergency rooms. This woman had real and present needs that, to me, were the fault of a failed system. This is what I had signed up for—helping the most vulnerable. It was why I had been drawn to this work, despite the challenges. It had meaning for me.

At the private hospital, although the patients presented as polite and well spoken, I also experienced a certain level of disrespect; it was just a lot more subtle and insidious. I could sense as soon as I entered a room if my white patients were going to have problems with me; I had learned to detect a flicker of confusion in their eyes as they sized me up, trying to figure out how I fit in. Who was this Black woman in a white coat? Was she the transporter? The nurse? The EKG technician? If yes, then why was she wearing the coat? The look in their eyes read, "Something is off here; something doesn't compute." Many times, I felt as if I was being interrogated for the job of physician by a white patient who wanted to make sure I was adequately trained.

"Where did you go to college?" people wanted to know.

"I went to Harvard," I'd reply.

"Oh, but where did you go to medical school?" they'd say.

"Harvard."

That usually ended the conversation, but it aggravated me that I had to justify my qualifications. I doubted any of my white colleagues had to do the same.

Some supposed misunderstandings became almost routine.

One time, the chief of service in the emergency department called to tell me there was a problem with one of my patients.

"Really?" I asked. "What's going on?"

The chief explained that this patient had complained he hadn't seen the supervising doctor yet.

"But I was just with that patient," I explained. "I saw him, examined him, and recommended treatment."

It didn't take us long to figure out what had happened. Although I had spent a full twenty minutes with this patient, this white man had refused to believe that a Black woman could be his supervising doctor.

Another time, I was taking care of an older white man with abdominal pain. I told him he needed an ultrasound right away.

"Okay, but I'd like to see that other doctor again," the patient said. "The one I saw before you got here, to make sure he agrees with you."

The doctor he had seen before me was my white male resident.

"Sir," I explained calmly, "I am the attending physician. This is a teaching hospital. That person you saw before me is still in training; I supervise him. He's here under my medical license. Every patient he sees I also have to see, and the decision about your care is ultimately up to me. He's a resident, whereas I am a practicing physician."

As time went on, I began to realize that patients like this man were genuinely unsettled by my presence. Why? Instinctively they were uncomfortable with the reality of a Black woman taking care of them. Not only that, I was a Black woman in a position of authority. My very presence within this private hospital had disrupted the status quo. Perhaps in order to regain power over the situation—when they were already feeling vulnerable and uncomfortable due to being in an emergency situation—these patients seemed determined to act in ways that undermined me.

One night, I had been on my shift for nearly eight hours and was getting ready to go home. My last visit was to a woman with pain in her calf. She had come to the ER with her daughter. After I'd examined the patient and told her it was a sprained muscle, the daughter asked me for a second opinion.

"And it's not because you're Black," she added.

It had been a tough shift and I was exhausted. All I wanted to do was to go home. But now I had to arrange for a second opinion demanded by my patient's daughter.

I asked my colleague, a white woman, to go and take a look. She came back and said, "I completely agree with you, it's a strained muscle."

That night as I left the ER, I felt angry. I was overcome by a wave of nausea, my cheeks were flushed, and I was on the verge of tears. I should have been home already, and instead, I'd had to stay to deal with a patient's daughter who wasn't satisfied with the diagnosis I had given her mother but "not because" of the color of my skin.

This was twenty-first-century New York City. No one hung signs over the doors of the Tisch and Bellevue saying COLOREDS and WHITES, but even so, these white patients sensed that somehow I must have walked in through the wrong door.

***

I believe that everyone who worked at Bellevue and Tisch knew that we were operating within a system of segregated care. Although my white colleagues might have liked to think that they were colorblind, they simply needed to use their eyes to see how the waiting rooms at the two emergency rooms stood in stark contrast to each other. Simply put, our patients were divided up based on insurance status and race. We saw mainly white patients at the private hospital and mainly patients of color at the public one. Period. The numbers bore this out. To this day, only 9 percent of the discharged patients at Tisch are Black, compared with 26 percent from Bellevue. The segregation was never acknowledged by the powers that be; it was accepted as the way things were. Acknowledging the differences would mean admitting there were deep systemic inequities in our society that desperately needed to be addressed. No one wanted to rock that boat.

Across the nation, studies show that Black patients are two to three times less likely than white patients to be seen at private academic medical centers, which have a reputation for providing superior care. Uninsured patients are five times less likely than patients with private insurance to be seen at these types of hospitals. What is true of New York is true of all the major metropolitan cities, Philadelphia, Boston, Detroit, LA, and Cleveland included. A recent study found that even in the eleven states that expanded Medicaid under the Affordable Care Act, patients of color were still more likely to use safety-net hospitals than non-safety-net hospitals, which have more specialists and resources. Even when a top-ranked non-safety-net hospital is located in the middle of a Black community, as is the case of the renowned Cleveland Clinic in Ohio, its patients can still skew predominantly white. Because of systemic racism, we have ended up with a two-tiered system in this country that contributes to bad outcomes for our most vulnerable patients and ends up costing us more in the long run. And everywhere in the US we accept this medical apartheid as the norm.

Working at NYU, we knew that when EMS picked up unhoused patients in an ambulance, they would never bring those patients to the private hospital. They only brought them to the public hospital. This was the unspoken rule. We all knew that interns weren't allowed to work at Tisch ER because that would mean a wealthy private patient might complain of inadequate care. Instead, if you were an intern, you went to work at the Bellevue ER, where the assumption was that people would be grateful for your help, no matter how inexperienced you were. If you made a mistake, it might go unnoticed, or at least no one would complain. These differences even translated to the clothing we wore. At Tisch, we were told as physicians we should always wear our white coats and a nice blouse or shirt, never scrubs; the assumption being that we needed to signal to our patients that we were qualified physicians. At Bellevue, there were no rules against wearing scrubs, with the assumption being that no one would notice or it didn't matter.

In my ten years working at Tisch and Bellevue, I can count on one hand the number of times anyone broke the silence about the existing segregated system of health care. When someone did, it was usually a Black person or person of color.

"How come the FDNY guys are so rude to the patients they bring to the ER at Bellevue?" one of my residents, Kamini, an Indo-Caribbean woman, asked one night. "They would never speak that way to a Tisch patient!"

She was right. The paramedics would routinely shout at the

public hospital patients and treat them roughly, while remaining courteous with the private patients in their care. The basic understanding was that it was okay to treat Bellevue patients like this, but it was not okay for Tisch patients.

Another time, Kamini railed against the different waiting times at the two hospitals.

"Why do Bellevue patients have to wait hours for care, whereas Tisch patients are seen within minutes?" Again, she was right. Waiting times were yet another example of the stark disparities in care.

For Kamini, all of this was personal. She had grown up in an uninsured immigrant family in a Caribbean neighborhood in Queens. Her whole family had relied on emergency rooms as their primary source of health care. In a rare quiet moment on one of our shifts, Kamini confided in me that she had once been driving in a car with her cousin when they were hit by an intoxicated driver. Their car lost control and hit a tree.

"When we were taken into an ambulance, the first question the EMS guy asked me was did I have an insurance card," Kamini remembered. When she couldn't show proof of insurance, she was taken to the public safety-net hospital that was miles away, instead of the private hospital that was right around the corner. "That was my first experience of segregated care," she told me. "After that, it was very clear that medicine was political."

After graduating college, Kamini had worked as a community organizer in East Harlem with Doctors for America, before deciding to go to medical school. During her training, she observed how communities like hers were seen by people in power as "wastelands waiting to be saved," as she described it. She became part of a broader social and racial justice movement, advocating for our communities to be supported in terms of resources and opportunities. She saw clearly our health-care system's lack of regard for Black people, especially in the ways it prioritized white people's lives and profit. And while I saw the problem too and had hoped that I could contribute to positive change through my leadership and presence at the institution, it was driving Kamini directly into advocacy and activism—in opposition to the hospital administration.

From my earliest days at NYU, my experience was so different from the one I'd had at Kings County. Working within my community, in an under-resourced setting, had left me physically and psychologically exhausted—but even as burned out as I was, my heart hadn't wanted to leave. I still felt an overwhelming love for my patients. I still felt an obligation to my community. I felt like I was a part of Kings County and Kings County was a part of me. In contrast, the minute I set foot in NYU, I knew in my bones that I would never experience the same feeling of belonging. I always felt disconnected. It didn't matter how friendly or accepting my colleagues were, the institution had always been clear about who mattered (or didn't) to them. After all, I was one of only two Black faculty members on staff in my department of more than one hundred faculty. This brought with it a different kind of exhaustion. Although we had far more resources at NYU than at Kings County, it could never feel like home.

At these ERs in the same city, I experienced firsthand deep inequities in our health-care system—one that is separate and unequal, with patients being divided up based on insurance and race. I thought about Kamini and other people who look like me that are living this segregated nightmare every day. Why should it fall solely on them to have to call out when something is so profoundly wrong? What would the hospitals in this city, and by extension this country, look like if we protected our most vulnerable and underserved communities and identified a pathway to ensuring single-payer, universal health care for every single person in the United States? How then might we break the cycles of trauma and injustice? These were the questions I was beginning to ask myself as my tenure at NYU went on.

NINE

Motherhood

I had been at NYU for three years when Chris and I decided to get married. We had a small wedding ceremony with family and friends at Brooklyn Botanic Garden next to the pond in the Japanese garden, my mother's favorite place in Brooklyn and the site where we had scattered her ashes sixteen years before. The choice of location for our ceremony was important to me: I wanted to feel my mother's presence at my wedding. It was a beautiful, blue-skied sunny day at the beginning of September, the light dappling our faces through the leaves of the maple trees, reflecting back from the water. I wore a simple white dress and a white fascinator in my hair. Chris's cousin—a judge—married us, and our guests stood in a circle around us as Chris and I read our vows. I didn't have a bridal party; just Oni, my maid of honor, but she was more than enough. As part of the ceremony, our aunt Joanie, my mother's only sister, sang one of my mother's favorite songs, "Moon River."

Shortly after getting married, Chris and I decided to start

trying for a baby. That November, I turned thirty-six, and to my surprise, the first time we tried, I got pregnant. I took a home pregnancy test, watching the little window for the double blue lines, holding my breath, then raced to call Chris to tell him the news. I felt a total sense of elation. Since my mother's death, there had been only a handful of times when I had felt this happy: at my medical school graduation, on my wedding day, and now, knowing that there was this new life growing inside me.

My joy at the news of becoming a mother was immediate. But the pleasure was soon tempered by my anxiety around pregnancy itself. Since my near-death experience with appendicitis as a student, I had done everything I could to stay out of the hospital as a patient. After I became pregnant, I knew I was going to have to interact with the medical system as a patient again, and I was not happy about it. I was a physician; you would think that my insider knowledge would have given me a sense of security. In fact, the opposite was true. Knowing everything I know about health care and the way we are treated as Black people, I had come to the conclusion that I simply couldn't get sick. It was just too dangerous for me to be anything apart from healthy.

But here I was, pregnant and in need of care. The fact is, as a Black birthing person with a college degree, I'm still five times more likely to die in childbirth than a white birthing person with the same qualifications. Even though I have excellent insurance, education, and access to quality care, the hard truth is that inequitable maternal health outcomes for Black birthing people persist across socioeconomic backgrounds and educational levels. My own mother had suffered with preeclampsia during her pregnancy (which can lead to serious and even fatal complications if untreated) and was forced to go on bed rest for the last two months before giving birth to my sister and me. My sister had miscarried her first pregnancy and had a C-section with her second, along with a difficult recovery. A little while before I learned I was pregnant, a close physician friend—a Black woman—who was young, in good health, and one year below me in residency, had returned to work after a short maternity leave experiencing very bad headaches, only to learn she had a brain bleed, a very rare complication of childbirth, which meant she had to have surgery to drain the blood. She ended up in the ICU and out of work for weeks recovering. It was a life-threatening event that thankfully she survived. Even US Representative Cori Bush has spoken about experiencing severe pain while pregnant with her first child, and when she described her symptoms to her physician, her concerns were swiftly dismissed. She ended up going into early labor a week later, at twenty-three weeks, and delivering a baby boy weighing 1 pound, 3 ounces. Though I had not yet heard Representative Bush's story, the message to me was clear: a Black birthing person who is otherwise healthy can have poor outcomes during pregnancy, childbirth, or postpartum.

With my growing focus on emergency ultrasound in my ER work, I inevitably ended up seeing many failed pregnancies in my work too. At Kings County in particular, these tended to be Black birthing people who would arrive early in pregnancy, bleeding or experiencing abdominal pain. Oftentimes I would finish a scan and have to tell a patient that they were miscarrying their baby or that I didn't detect a heartbeat at a point in the pregnancy when I should have been able to. It was heartbreaking. As my patients shed tears, I bore witness firsthand to the toll that's placed on Black birthing people by systemic racism (and sexism)—the stress and socioeconomic disadvantages that are so deep and rampant that they affect every aspect of how we experience maternity and motherhood in this country.

The statistics are staggering. To this day, the United States spends more on health care and births than any other country in the world, but it also has one of the highest maternal mortality rates of any high-income nation. These numbers are in large part driven by the high Black maternal mortality rate, with Black birthing people three to four times more likely to die of pregnancy-related complications than white birthing people. In NYC, where I was born, raised, and live, the Black maternal mortality rate is nine times as high as it is for their white peers. When compared with white birthing people, Black birthing people in the United States are twice as likely to have a preterm birth, give birth to a low-birth-weight baby, or have a child that dies before the age of one. Contributing to the problem is the fact that health-care professionals often dismiss Black birthing people's health concerns. A survey from 2019 that polled birthing people of all races showed that more than 22 percent of Black birthing people reported mistreatment by a health-care professional during their pregnancies and childbirth. It also showed that birthing people of color are twice as likely as their white peers to report being ignored by a health-care professional when they reported symptoms or asked for help.

What could I do with this kind of information but register it and then set it aside, doing my best to reassure myself that I was going to be okay as a patient? To be a Black birthing person in this country and to bring new life into the world—despite the dangers, despite the risks, despite systemic racism—are acts of resistance. My mother would have known this truth, just as generations of Black parents have understood it. You make a conscious decision to love and be loved, to grow your family, despite the incredible odds stacked against you and your children. While others in positions of more privilege may take starting a family for granted, you have to insist on your right to do so, accepting all the happiness and pain that might come with the territory.

I went into my first pregnancy with a sense of trepidation and caution, as if on tiptoe. I didn't tell a lot of people I was pregnant in the early stages, hiding my growing bump under my loose scrubs and oversize white coat. My obstetrician-gynecologist (ob-gyn) ended up being a white woman born in Italy who had a small practice that was affiliated with NYU. Her practice was recommended to me by one of my Black physician assistant friends, who reported a reassuring and positive birthing experience. Although I didn't end up going with an ob-gyn who was Black—because the doctor I chose delivered in the same building where I worked, and I wanted that convenience—I did make sure she would listen to me and understand my concerns. I didn't want to be dismissed. I wanted to feel properly supported. I mostly appreciated that this ob-gyn's practice was known and recommended for its low C-section rate and was highly utilized by resident and attending physicians at NYU. A C-section can increase the risk of mortality for the birthing person. The reality is that Black birthing people are 36 percent more likely to have a C-section than birthing people of other races.

"You have to be strong and healthy to labor," my ob-gyn told me in her thick Italian accent at my first appointment. "You can start working on that now."

This was what I wanted to hear: that there was something I could do to control my chances of a safe pregnancy and delivery. As my pregnancy progressed, I found I looked forward to visiting my ob-gyn's office, with the pictures of all the babies she had delivered pinned to the walls. But despite the care of my compassionate ob-gyn, the privileges of my education, not to mention my excellent insurance, I still worried about how much I was worrying. I thought a lot about weathering during my pregnancy, how internalizing the external stress of everyday racism manifests itself in our bodies. Research shows that the stress a birthing person goes through during pregnancy can have a hormonal impact on the baby, even leading to diabetes for the child later in life. Black birthing people are also more likely to go into preterm labor, to have premature babies, and to have babies with low birth weights. We're more likely to have pregnancy-induced hypertension. Preeclampsia, the condition from which my mother suffered when she was pregnant with my sister and me, is 60 percent more common in Black birthing people than in their white counterparts. Of course, I was worried about the effect that stress would have on my health and on our baby, especially as I worked in such a demanding and intense specialty, working eight-hour shifts in which I was mostly on my feet. I did what I could. I took care of myself as I had promised the ob-gyn I would and as my mother had always taught me to do, eating nutritious foods, exercising, trying to rest as much as possible when I wasn't working.

As with most people experiencing pregnancy for the first time, everything felt both surreal and awe-inspiring. I found out early through a blood test—because I was over thirty-five years old and considered to be of advanced maternal age—that we were having a boy. My initial reaction was bemusement. I hadn't grown up around many boys in our family. What was I going to do with a son? Thankfully, the answer came to me immediately: "You will love him." Around fourteen weeks into the pregnancy, I felt the fluttering inside me called quickening, the first palpable indication of the life I was carrying. The sound of the heartbeat at my prenatal checkups was further evidence of this growing person taking shape inside me. I was accustomed to seeing ultrasound images thanks to my emergency ultrasound expertise, but even so, the first time seeing my baby on-screen, those little smudges of white and gray on a black background, I felt overcome with emotion. The sense of tenderness and protectiveness for this human being was overwhelming. Who would he turn out to be? Later in pregnancy, feeling our baby kicking inside me gave me comfort despite my anxiety.

Not a day went by during my pregnancy that I didn't think of my mother and how she might have counseled and supported me if she had been here. Unlike me, she had struggled to conceive, eventually taking a fertility pill to help, which she knew increased her chances of giving birth to multiples. When she learned she was having twins, her initial reaction was simply relief that she didn't have triplets. It still amazes me that she chose to become a parent during her residency in internal medicine at Harlem Hospital. She was working incredibly long shifts, under tremendous pressure, in a woefully under-resourced environment. In the essay she wrote the year before she died, she recalled, "My first night on call after my return was the worst. I missed my baby daughters Oni and Uché very much. I wanted to give it all up and go home and just be a mother. But each night spent on call got better, and the horrible, terrible, empty, aching feeling lessened." Although there were times during my pregnancy when I wondered how I was going to be able to juggle a family and a career, I knew I only had to look to her example. As a child, it was clear to me that my mother's work was her calling; I also knew that she loved me completely, and without question—I never felt neglected or ignored. Quite the contrary, my sister and I always felt showered with love and affection by our mother. Although I know now as an adult that she struggled with striking the right balance (if it is even possible!) between work and home as most women do, her career and her mothering always felt completely compatible to me. Yet again, her role-modeling was extending across the years even with her physical absence.

Thankfully, despite all my concerns during my pregnancy, I carried our baby to full term without major complications. He was born safely, which isn't to say that the experience wasn't a grueling one. I labored for seventeen hours before I was ready to push, and after that, I ended up pushing for another six full hours, breaking blood vessels in my eyes, my face becoming horribly swollen from the effort. Eventually my ob-gyn decided to do an episiotomy, so she could use forceps to get the baby out. Although

Chris was present and very supportive, I would have done anything to have my mother there with me, just to hear her tell me, "You can do this," as she used to do every time I faced a challenge.

Once our baby was finally out, I remember anxiously asking the ob-gyn, "Is he okay, is he okay?" I could hear him crying, which I knew was a good sign. The ob-gyn checked him out, then the nurses took him to the warmer to stimulate him and clean him off. Then they gave him to me, wrapped up in his swaddling cloth, telling me he was healthy and fine. It was the sweetest moment, lying there with my child on my chest, my heart on the outside of my body. I stroked his tiny head, looking into his eyes for the first time, promising him I would give him my all.

Recovering from childbirth was much harder than I had anticipated, however. Although I'd had an epidural, I still had intense pain radiating down my right leg throughout my labor. Two days after the delivery, I realized I couldn't feel the bottom of my right foot. When it came time to check out of the hospital, I stopped the ob-gyn who was covering for my doctor and said, "I'm having numbness on the bottom of my right foot—is this going to go away? I'm really worried."

She brushed off my concerns, saying, "Oh yes, you'll be fine," as she signed the paperwork and briskly left the room, leaving no time for further discussion.

Although the numbness in my foot did eventually go away after several weeks, I was left feeling unsettled by that ob-gyn's dismissive response to my concern. The prolonged pushing had caused the neuropathy. But what had caused me to push for six hours? I began to question a lot of things about my labor and delivery. Could the less-than-ideal forceps and episiotomy have been avoided?

Chris went back to work only a few weeks after our child was born, and I found myself at home alone with the baby. I had no real support during the day. I didn't have my mother, and my sister had her own small child and a demanding job.

When it came to breastfeeding, I immediately struggled to get him to latch properly, experiencing extreme pain each time I nursed him. If my mother had been there, perhaps she could have shown me the proper technique, as she did breastfeed us for a short period. Breastfeeding rates are quite low for Black birthing people across socioeconomic status, and of all groups, we are the least likely to nurse, for multiple reasons related to systemic racism. In part, this is because there tend to be far fewer baby-friendly hospitals to offer lactation support and resources to encourage breastfeeding in Black neighborhoods. Black women are more likely to be uninsured or to have Medicaid as their health insurance, but Medicaid has not been expanded in twelve states, which have large Black populations, and out-of-pocket costs for lactation consultants can be prohibitive for many. Black birthing people often face increased economic pressures to return to the workplace sooner, and they're less likely to work in jobs that offer the kind of flexibility that comes with paid family leave and allows them time to be at home with a newborn. What's more, Black birthing people may have conflicting feelings about breastfeeding, based on the ways our bodies have historically been sexualized or commodified, not to mention the deep trauma of slavery, in which enslaved women were forced to wet-nurse their enslavers' babies. All these cultural, societal, and historical forces conspire to make breastfeeding a complex choice for Black birthing people, when all birthing people should be supported in making the best decision for themselves when it comes to breastfeeding. I knew I was fortunate to be able to afford a lactation consultant, who helped me learn to latch the baby properly. Without her, I'm certain I would have stopped nursing during those first few weeks, unable to withstand the discomfort of it.

During those lonely weeks postpartum I thought about how after Oni and I were born, my mother called on our grandmother, our aunt, and our uncles to help out. In most African cultures, the family lives together—you always have extended family around, helping out, showing you how to nurse and care for the baby. By contrast, I felt isolated. The recovery from the episiotomy meant I couldn't sit down while the incision was healing, and it took about eight weeks to get back to normal. I experienced some postpartum blues—which is common due to the change in hormones, factoring in lack of sleep and not having a lot of family support. I still hungered for someone to mother me, even now that I was a mother myself. While pregnant, I'd wondered if becoming a mom would take me one step closer to healing from the loss of my mother, but now that our baby was here, I found I missed her even more.

It was during this difficult time that I remember a friend asking me if I'd ever considered hiring a doula to help me cope.

"A doula?" I asked. "What's that?"

Today, doulas are seen as one of the primary solutions that policy-makers recommend in addressing the Black maternal mortality crisis, and there is good data to show that they can improve outcomes in birthing people and babies, especially when combined with other kinds of support and care. Back in 2014, when I first gave birth, however, doulas just weren't on my own radar. The term is of ancient Greek origin, meaning "a woman who serves," and was popularized in the 1970s by Dana Louise Raphael, a US medical anthropologist who believed in the vital importance of breastfeeding and of nonmedical caregivers before, during, and after childbirth. The idea of a doula is that this person "mothers the mother," taking some of the stress out of what can be an intimidating experience for most birthing people. When you have a doula, you have someone to advocate for you, to ask the right questions, and to be there for you in all phases of your pregnancy, labor, and postpartum. In Black communities, doulas are especially critical in providing culturally responsive care and support that can be invaluable to Black birthing people, especially when there are so few Black ob-gyns. There is evidence to suggest that continuous support during childbirth, such as the type of support that doulas provide, can increase the chance of a vaginal delivery and decrease the likelihood of C-section and instrumental birth, like I had during my first delivery. It can also reduce the need for epidural anesthesia and increase the rate of breastfeeding, which substantially improves the health of new mothers and babies.

While the term *doula* is relatively new, the role is as old as time, especially in Black communities. Black women have always supported one another around pregnancy, childbirth, and parenting, whether as grandmothers, aunties, sisters, friends, or birth workers. In fact, there is a long rich history of Black birth workers that is rarely acknowledged in the medical literature. During the seventeenth century, when enslaved Africans were first brought to these shores by European colonists, there would have been women among them who knew how to care for pregnant and laboring people, and who brought their traditional birth practices with them. These women passed down their knowledge from generation to generation, their descendants going on to do the work of midwives, doulas, and lactation experts long before there were terms to describe these roles. During the Jim Crow era in the South, when many hospitals denied access to Black women, Black "Granny midwives," as they were known, traveled from house to house making sure that Black mothers received the care they needed, no matter where they lived or how much they could afford to pay. These midwives were pillars of their communities, well known and respected.

That all changed after the turn of the twentieth century, when the 1910 Flexner Report—which made recommendations for the standardization of medical institutions and practices that led to the closures of historically Black medical schools—radically changed the landscape of birth workers too. Midwives with decades of experience found that in order to practice legally, they had to fulfill certain requirements and training that only white women had access to or were able to afford. Across the board, public health reforms and the rise of physician-attended births led to the medicalization of pregnancy and childbirth; births shifted from the home setting into hospitals. In 1921, the Sheppard-Towner Act initiated a campaign to portray midwives as unqualified and as the contributing factor to high maternal and infant mortality rates. The funds from this act were directed to state health departments for midwife training programs and led to even stricter guidelines and certification requirements. Midwives in general began to be sidelined, regarded as old-fashioned and unsafe, even though these perceptions were far from accurate. In fact, a New York Academy of Medicine study in 1932 found that home births attended by midwives had the lowest maternal mortality rates of any setting. Despite this, ob-gyns and the medicalized model of managing pregnancy and childbirth became the norm.

In 1900, the United States had 100,000 midwives who attended 50 percent of all births. At the time of the writing of this book, there are only 15,000 midwives in this country, and fewer than 1,000 are Black; midwives attend only 8 percent of all births. An abundance of studies show that out-of-hospital births are associated with lower C-section and maternal mortality rates and that if we increased midwife-delivered births, we could actually avert 40 percent of maternal deaths. Midwifery has been shown to reduce the use of medical interventions such as epidurals and C-sections, which are associated with greater risks than vaginal deliveries. In 2018, however, nearly 40 percent of all deliveries in the US were by C-section—which increases the risk of illness and death for birthing people—even though the World Health Organi-

zation recommends that the rate should be closer to 10 to 15 percent. Meanwhile, a full 98 percent of US births currently take
place in hospitals, even though 85 percent of birthing people in
the US are considered low-risk and would qualify for an out-of-
hospital birth if they had the option. Black birthing people have
greater barriers to access and fewer choices for maternity care
that meets their needs. For example, 69 percent of Black respon-
dents to the 2013 Listening to Mothers survey were interested in
having an out-of-hospital birth, but only if they could find a maternity care clinician who shared their cultural identity and experience. Perhaps more calculating and disturbing have been the
financial incentives, in terms of insurance reimbursement, that
helped to turn birthing into and sustain it as a medicalized and
hospitalized procedure that generates revenue.

Two years after our first child was born, when I learned I was
pregnant for a second time, I did decide I needed more emotional
support and that I wanted to hire a doula. I went online, got referrals, and interviewed five different women—all Black. I felt incredibly fortunate to find the number of potential doula candidates I
did, especially because a 2003 study found that most doulas at
the time were white, well-educated, married women with children.
For many doulas of color, their primary motivation for doing birth
work is to support women from their own racial, ethnic, and cultural community. I immediately connected with one of the doula
candidates and chose to work with her right away. She was a kind
and warm woman a few years younger than me who already had

five children of her own. She understood the dynamics of what happens to a Black birthing person in the hospital during labor—how easy it is for us to be dismissed, our concerns minimized, our pain ignored. I felt comforted knowing she was going to be there for me. The cost of a doula can range from four hundred to thirty-five hundred dollars for a delivery, and these costs are often not covered by insurance. I knew it was a privilege to be able to afford these services, and that the price of a doula is prohibitive for many Black birthing people because most of us make fourteen cents less on the dollar than white women, and 70 percent of us are the primary breadwinners in our homes.

During my second pregnancy I met regularly with my doula to talk about how I wanted the birth to go. We practiced different breathing techniques and I learned natural ways to make labor more bearable. I was shaken up from my first experience of childbirth and hoped not to repeat it. The fact that my doula was going to be there, that she was knowledgeable and would advocate for me, helped soothe my nerves.

My second labor was not without its own drama, but it was ultimately safe and swift. Shortly after my arrival at the labor and delivery ward, the nurse told me she was having a difficult time detecting the baby's heartbeat via the tocodynamometer. After she tried a few times and couldn't hear anything, I became distraught. Fortunately, my doula was there throughout, to hold my hand, to reassure me. I was rushed to OR, where it was assumed I would need a C-section. As it turned out, the reason we couldn't hear the heartbeat was that my labor was progressing so quickly that the baby was much lower in the birth canal than anyone expected. I pushed three times, and out he came. The entire labor was only five hours. My doula stayed with me at the hospital, making sure I ate and drank, that I was well tended to, that the baby latched well. In the weeks after I came home, she would visit regularly to help me out, making meals and entertaining our elder child. It was a big difference from my first time, when I had felt so very lonely. Clearly, not every Black birthing person in this country is as lucky as I was to give birth to two babies safely and without major incident—and with the support of a lactation consultant and doula.

Black birthing people are still dying in childbirth in terrifying numbers. Every now and again, these stories make the news, like that of Dr. Chaniece Wallace, a Black pediatrician in Indianapolis, who died in 2020 due to preeclampsia complications two days after she welcomed her daughter into the world. Or Sha-Asia Washington, a teacher's aide from Brooklyn who, the same year, died of cardiac arrest just two hours after delivering a healthy baby girl via C-section. In a well-resourced country such as ours, the death of any birthing person from preventable conditions should be nothing short of a national scandal. And yet Black birthing people still die in the hundreds every single year.

As I write this, the Black maternal health crisis has reached such a peak that legislative action is finally taking place to address it. Work is being done by the Black Maternal Health Caucus, led by Representative Lauren Underwood, a registered nurse herself. Underwood's efforts have focused on advancing the Black Maternal Health Momnibus Act of 2021, which contains twelve individual bills to comprehensively address this crisis. The act acknowledges that doulas are part of the solution to high Black maternal mortality rates, and that addressing the problem is both complex and complicated because racism manifests both overtly and covertly. Some of the policy solutions address the impact of the social determinants of health on maternal health outcomes by investing in housing, transportation, and access to health foods for Black birthing people. Other bills focus on providing support and funding for diversifying the perinatal workforce, because increasing the number of Black birth workers would likely have a positive impact on maternal and infant health outcomes. There are even policies calling for investments in data collection processes and quality measures to better understand the factors that lead to the high Black maternal mortality rate. Another policy focuses on investing in telehealth and other digital tools to improve maternal health outcomes in rural and other underserved areas.

As momentum increases to address this crisis in earnest, the good news is that there are models out there that have shown success in improving outcomes for Black birthing people and their babies—and they are rooted in the work of doulas and midwives who recognize the need for holistic support for families. A 2019 study of a Black-owned, midwife-led freestanding birth center in north Minneapolis, for example, shows how a community-centered model of care can reduce health disparities and even costs. The Roots Community Birth Center is located in a majority Black, low-income neighborhood. Its staff—which includes midwives, doulas, and family physicians—offers out-of-hospital births tailored to the individual needs of each birthing person. They practice culturally centered care, which is to say that they seek to understand and respect the values held by their patients and rec-ognize the systemic factors that contribute to their pregnancy and birthing experience. Over the four years of the study, Roots had zero preterm births, even though Black birthing people in the United States are twice as likely to have a preterm birth than white birthing people, and even though the center is located in a neighborhood with the highest infant mortality rate in Minneapolis. Essentially, the Roots model shows that simply recognizing a Black birthing person's humanity while providing care can make a tremendous impact on maternal and infant health outcomes.

Community-based birth centers like these are combating the racial inequities that exist within maternal and child health—but they are few and far between. We need more of them. The women running these centers are playing their part in challenging and dismantling the systems of racism and patriarchy, just as Black birth workers did in the past as they traveled from house to house, caring for their communities, nurturing parents and the next generation alike.

Looking back, it's interesting to me that as anxious as I was during my pregnancies, I had never even considered an out-of-hospital birth. I had been socialized, educated, and trained within the biomedical model of Western medicine. I had always assumed that an ob-gyn would care for me during my pregnancies and that I would give birth to my children within a hospital setting. I didn't know the history of Black midwives or the benefits of the out-of-hospital birthing model. Once I did, I mourned what my birthing experiences could have been.

TEN

Diversity and Exclusion

I spotted Natasha as soon as I walked into the room: a young Black student nervously standing on her own, cocoa-complexioned with long box braids that reached down to her mid-back, with her arms folded close to her chest. We were both attending a meet and greet held in a conference room at NYU School of Medicine. The school's Office of Diversity Affairs sponsored the event to welcome new Black, Latinx, and Native American students at the beginning of the academic year. I, along with the other Black faculty and faculty of color, had been invited, and as there were so few of us at NYU, I made sure to attend. Just the sight of Natasha standing on her own made me want to run over to her. I could remember the many times as a student and even as faculty that I'd felt out of place, out of my comfort zone.

After introducing myself and exchanging pleasantries, I got straight to the point: "Natasha, I'd really like to mentor you." A look of relief flashed across her face, and we agreed to meet the next week for coffee.

Natasha was one of the first students I developed a real connection with at NYU, and we stayed in close contact throughout her time at the school. From day one in my new job, I felt that my role as a faculty member was more than just a career move. It was about transforming a space that had historically and intentionally excluded us, a way of redressing the legacy of institutional racism, effectively changing the color of the faces on the Hall of Portraits with my presence. Most of the leadership roles in the department were held by much older white men, and although my new colleagues were friendly and seemed to treat me as a peer, I took note that none of them even acknowledged or mentioned the fact that we had only two Black faculty in the entire Department of Emergency Medicine. Academic medical centers, like NYU, are the premier places where medical students learn how to become physicians and where faculty members engage in cutting-edge education, research, and clinical care. My mindset was that in order to make a difference as a Black woman in medicine, it was going to be necessary for me to carve out a path within an institution like this one, creating a more inclusive space for Black students and faculty, so that I could ultimately reach a position of influence where I could actually bring about real systemic change.

Another big reason I had wanted to stay at an academic institution was because I loved to teach and interact with students and residents like Natasha. I felt a responsibility to them. It's now well established that the route to success in academic medicine is through a successful mentor. Your mentors create a road map for you and give you opportunities such as being a part of a research project or coauthoring papers, which can lead to recognition and promotions. Studies show the positive impact mentorship can have not just on medical students, but on entire institutions, when mentoring is valued. Yet research also shows that people are more likely to choose mentors who look like them—and so when you have a department with only a handful of faculty of color, there are few faculty members to effectively mentor the students of color. This is not just a problem at NYU. A recent study revealed that across the country, medical school faculty are almost 63.9 percent white and 58.6 percent male, especially at the professor and associate levels—but at NYU the numbers were even more dismal than at other academic medical centers.

For my part, I wanted to be someone's role model because I knew what it was like to navigate medical school with hardly any people of color on faculty to look up to. Even after I arrived at NYU, I had to search high and low for a mentor of my own, eventually finding an older white woman in internal medicine who agreed to help me. I wasn't even faculty in her department, but she was someone who cared deeply about equity and justice. She was very aware of how sexism had reared its ugly head in academic medicine, and she was empathic enough to see how racism had negatively affected her Black colleagues. We would meet every few months. Our meetings would always start with me sitting down with a grin on my face, saying, "I'm meeting with my chair next week and I need your help . . . again." She'd always give me a tender but confident smile and say, "Of course, Uché. I'm here for you."

During those meetings, we would discuss how I should go about negotiating my protected time. In academia, the goal is to have nonclinical time to focus and develop your academic interests, but it was already hard to come by this protected time, as it's known, because the departments were quite stingy with their funds, and you had to work hard to prove yourself worthy first. My mentor had been successful at navigating the world of academic medicine and would happily share her wisdom with me to increase my chances of a successful negotiation with my chair. During our meetings, I felt safe sharing my concerns about how few Black people there were in leadership roles within the institution. In time, she would leave NYU, and what a profound loss it was. She had hit that point that it seems every brilliant woman gets to, where the men around her feel threatened and there aren't any opportunities for growth. I was grateful to have had at least one person who took a vested interest in my career development.

In turn, I made sure to meet up regularly with my new mentee, Natasha, to chat and check in. I learned she was born and raised in New Jersey, that her family was from Jamaica, and she was a first-generation American and the first in her family to attend college. Natasha had gone through high school and college in New Jersey in classrooms with predominantly Black students, and so when she arrived at NYU and learned she was one of only six students of color in her class, it was a real shock to her system.

When we sat down for coffee together, her face looked pained and drawn.

"It's like I'm constantly questioning whether I belong here," she'd tell me, taking small bites of a pastry. "Even though I know

I've earned the right, I keep thinking I'm going to wake up one day and there's going to be an email from NYU saying they made some big mistake and that I don't really deserve to be here after all."

During her time at NYU, Natasha had to contend with a lot of pressures that most of her classmates did not have to worry about. She had family issues at home—her parents were divorced and the family was having a tough time financially. At one point her mother and younger brothers were evicted from their home. Even though she was receiving financial aid, Natasha was still struggling with affording her living expenses while helping her family with extra money when they needed it. While many of her wealthier classmates were spending the weekends vacationing in the Hamptons, she usually had to go home to New Jersey to help her mom and brothers. Thankfully, Natasha felt comfortable opening up to me—and with her permission I was able to discuss her situation with staff and faculty in the Office of Diversity Affairs to make sure they understood what she was going through.

One day, when her name was accidentally omitted from a group list for one of her classes, she told me that she took this as confirmation of her worst fears: "It's like now I finally have proof I'm not supposed to be here!"

As soon as those words rolled out of Natasha's mouth, I felt a pressure in my chest.

I knew I had to be honest with her.

"Natasha, I know how you feel. I've felt the same way. Many times. And sometimes I still do."

"What? Even you, Dr. Blackstock?" she replied, looking at me in disbelief.

At my department's monthly faculty meetings, I'd often look around at my one-hundred-plus colleagues and realize I was the only person who looked like me in the entire conference room. A hospital in the middle of New York City, one of the most diverse cities in the world, and yet I was often the only Black woman. Comments from a white colleague about how I often changed my hairstyle or another telling me excitedly how their child had be-friended a Black child in their class, as if they should receive an award for it, were constant reminders that I was different.

"Yes, even me," I told Natasha. "But we do belong here. We deserve to be here. I'm here to remind you of that," I said as I squeezed her hand gently.

My words were heartfelt, but in some ways disingenuous. I had to encourage her to keep going even though we were constantly made to feel that we didn't belong here. It felt like an unfair posi-tion to put her in, but it was our reality.

Natasha and I talked at length about impostor syndrome. The term has always rubbed me the wrong way. The fact is, like race, impostor syndrome is a social construct, and like race, it's a prod-uct of racism, sexism, and other systems of oppression that limit access to opportunities, resources, and power. For a lot of the time I spent with Natasha, I'd simply listen and validate for her that she was more than deserving and worthy, despite the evident chal-lenges. Many of her classmates came from wealthy, privileged backgrounds—some of them children of physicians who had con-stant guidance from their parents about how to navigate medical school—which only added to her sense of isolation.

Although her story was very different from mine, I'd also gone through school while navigating turbulent times at home, with the loss of my mother. Even though I was raised by a mother who was a physician, even though I studied my behind off, there were times I worried that I wasn't good enough, and that I wasn't going to be able to succeed, because I received constant reminders that I was different.

And of course, Natasha reminded me of my mom. Like Natasha, my mother had been the first in her family to go to college, and she too had felt lost and vulnerable at medical school, in an environment that wasn't designed with her in mind. In fact, it has been designed to intentionally exclude Black people like Natasha and me. There were so many moments when it would have been easy for my mother to drop out, yet she was determined to graduate, and so was Natasha.

Perhaps because of my mother's challenges as a young woman, she had always seen the potential in people and nurtured that. When she was at Kings County, she mentored a younger colleague who was a social worker, and who had aspirations of becoming a physician. They had many conversations in the hospital hallways, my mother prodding the young woman to take her postbaccalaureate classes and MCAT exam and apply to medical school. A few times the young woman even shadowed my mother while she saw her patients in the clinic. Eventually, she fulfilled all her medical school requirements, applied to medical school, and was accepted. My mother's mentee became a close family friend of ours and board-certified in physical and rehabilitation medicine.

Mentoring had been so important to my mother, and it became very important to me too.

In the fall of 2013—three years after I arrived at NYU and at the beginning of Natasha's third year—a ripple of outrage went out around the student body. Classes at the school had never been particularly diverse, but this year was far worse than usual. Out of the 206 incoming NYU medical students, only one was Black. Natasha had been one of six the year before, which is hardly a huge number but at least she wasn't "the only." The single Black student was Haitian American and from the same Afro-Caribbean neighborhood in Brooklyn where Kings County Hospital was located. Once I heard about her, I reached out to connect with her in person, meeting with her as often as time allowed to offer my support.

During her time at NYU, this student had made the best of things, but it was clear that the administration itself, outside of the Office of Diversity Affairs, was barely doing anything to provide her with extra support and resources. NYU needed to put more effort into recruiting a diverse student body, but instead, they weren't even acknowledging that there was a diversity problem. Again, this was indicative of a national problem, with Black and Latinx people currently making up about 31 percent of the population but comprising on average around 15 percent of first-year medical students. Sadly, the numbers at NYU in 2013 were well below national averages and among the lowest in the New York area.

Natasha shared my outrage.

"In the middle of New York, the most diverse city in the world, you mean to tell me there's only one Black student worthy of studying at NYU?" she asked. I pointed out that even when my mother had been at Harvard Medical School in the 1970s, she and other Black students made up 10 percent of her class.

Unlike the administration, Natasha was already taking action. Together with a fellow student, Aaron, they had connected with the first-year student and adopted her as a friend. And they had gone further than that, banding together with other student leaders to start the Student Diversity Initiative (SDI) to try to recruit a more diverse student body.

"Everyone needs to get involved in this," Natasha insisted. "We're going to pull people from all backgrounds; we need a concerted effort here. We need more students of color in this school."

In the coming months, Natasha spent hours reaching out to every person of color she could find among the NYU student body, staff, and faculty, getting them to rally around the initiative. Together with her friends, they created what became known as the SEED program—Supporting, Educating, and Enriching Diversity. The program's goal was to support students who were historically excluded and currently underrepresented in medicine by offering them structured mentoring while in medical school. First-year medical students were offered mentoring by groups of upper-year medical students, residents, and attending physicians known as "families." I was more than happy to serve as a SEED family member.

The following summer, we learned the horrific news of the Eric Garner killing in July 2014. His murder had taken place in broad daylight while he was trying to break up a fight. The police accosted him because they suspected he was selling loose cigarettes, which is considered a minor offense and was simply a way for Mr. Garner to earn money. Without poverty and racism, Mr. Garner would never have been put in that situation in the first place. He was handcuffed for a nonviolent offense, roughed up, and his pleas of "I can't breathe!" were ignored. I remember watching the video, my stomach in knots, thinking, "He's not breathing. . . . No one is helping him." The police and EMS workers didn't even consider him a human being. Afterward, the police and media implicated Mr. Garner in his own death, blaming his poor health, another consequence of racism and poverty. As I followed the story of Mr. Garner's murder, what gutted me even more was how his daughter Erica Garner, who fought so valiantly for justice for her father, ended up dying of a pregnancy-related complication: cardiomyopathy, a pregnancy-induced condition that is more common in Black birthing people than in white birthing people.

The month after Mr. Garner's killing, Michael Brown was shot in the back by police. I remember coming into work exhausted and angry, unable to think of anything else. As the day unfolded, I was shocked and infuriated that not a single white or non-Black colleague had commented on what had taken place. Thankfully, our students were much more vocal. Many of them excused themselves from classes to attend protests that were happening around the city in support of the protests in Ferguson, Missouri. They even organized a "die-in" in the lobby of Bellevue Hospital, where they all lay down on the floor in silence to draw attention to the twin crises of racism and police brutality. They had initially thought about holding the protest in the lobby of NYU's private hospital, Tisch, but they were concerned that they would get in trouble with the school's administration if they held the protest in a hospital where the patients were predominantly white and affluent. And so, they held their protest at Bellevue, the public hospital whose population was made up of Black, Latinx, immigrant, and unhoused patients.

After the protest, the students, especially those who made up the Student Diversity Initiative, called for a follow-up town hall meeting with school leaders. They wanted to talk about Ferguson and the ongoing issues of lack of diversity and inclusion at NYU. They decided that white students should speak on behalf of the students of color, so that students of color wouldn't be retaliated against or labeled as troublemakers by the administration. At the town hall, the white students went ahead and raised the students' concerns about bias and racism within the school. But instead of addressing these concerns, the medical school leaders were simply upset that the students had the gall to bring up what they considered controversial issues. After the town hall, the students were left with the impression that leadership didn't want them to be activists or to care about racism or social justice; they were there solely to do their academic work, without acknowledging the upheaval around them and across the nation.

These students did not plan to remain silent, however. They were informed. They were vocal. They were putting the fire under the administration's feet. They were asking a lot of questions. Why were we seeing these racial health inequities in our communities? Why weren't we talking about systemic racism explicitly in class? Why weren't they learning about forgotten figures such as Henrietta Lacks as part of the curriculum?

While I was incredibly proud of everything that Natasha and her classmates were achieving, at the same time I could see it was taking a toll. All this work was student-driven, with students taking time out of their academic schedules to run and manage everything from protests to community-building activities to professional-development sessions. At another one of our informal catch-ups over coffee, Natasha shared that she was feeling overwhelmed working on the upcoming Diversity Week, yet another initiative that she and other students had to start to create a more inclusive environment at NYU for current students of color.

"I barely slept last night," she shared, her eyes looking tired. "I was up until this morning finalizing the schedule and making sure that everything goes as planned." She took a deep breath and exhaled. "I'm worried I'm burning out," she said, sliding back into her seat. "I'm just not sure I can do this anymore."

I looked at her sympathetically. I felt both sad and angry for Natasha and her classmates. The fact was that all the diversity and inclusion efforts they were creating took hours and hours of their time and far more of their energy than any of their white classmates and faculty could ever know or understand. These students were actively recruiting more students of color to the school—and NYU was benefiting as a result. Yet there was no compensation, either tangible or intangible, to students running these initiatives. Instead, Natasha was doing this work on top of her academic workload and her responsibilities to her family, because she knew it would not get done otherwise. Medical school is intense enough without adding the extra burden of overhauling the systemic inequities of an institution that isn't supporting its Black and other students of color in the first place. Natasha should have been in medical school to focus on becoming a physician. Instead she was worn out trying to dismantle racism from the ground up.

The environment was also beginning to take its toll on me. By 2014, I was the only Black faculty member in my department. The only other Black faculty member during my years as an assistant professor had left NYU because he felt that he had hit the ceiling in terms of professional opportunities within the institution. When he was offered the opportunity to be a vice chair of emergency medicine at another hospital in the city, he left because he saw no future within our department or at the school in general. After he left, the loss was profound in many ways. For the students and residents, it was one less Black faculty member, out of an already tiny pool, to mentor them. In any given week, I wasn't meeting just with Natasha but with multiple students, who barely had anyone else to turn to who could understand their concerns and experiences. And just as Natasha wasn't being compensated for her time spearheading diversity initiatives, my involvement in mentoring her and other students was rarely appreciated or formally acknowledged by the institution. Needless to say, I had little protected time in my schedule for the important work of mentoring students.

On top of this, I was often asked to lead or be involved in diversity and inclusion efforts, such as participating on diversity committees within my department, within the medical school, or university-wide. Although I was rarely compensated in protected time or salary for this invaluable work, I always said yes. I knew the work was important, and I made sure to prepare carefully before each event. Yet, I found it ironic and infuriating that we, Black faculty members, were being given the complex and overwhelming task of remedying the outcomes of centuries of institutionalized racism—problems we did not create in the first place. The issue with doing the unpaid labor of diversity, equity, inclusion, and anti-racism is that it leaves you overwhelmed and with less time to do your other work. Like the inimitable Toni Morrison said in 1975, "The very serious function of racism is a distraction. It keeps you from doing your work." And in academia, there is a much higher value placed on how many journal articles you write, or how much research funding you bring into the school, than the number of students you mentor or how many diversity panels you serve on.

Ever since having my children, my life had understandably gone through an enormous shift. While I'd always had the time and flexibility to focus on my work, that time disappeared. Adding to that, the extra workload of mentoring students and contributing to the diversity push left me feeling like I wasn't doing a good job at either of my roles—mother or physician. As professional women, we put tremendous pressure on ourselves, as do our workplaces, loved ones, and society. For the first few years after having my children, I felt like I was barely keeping my head above water at work and at home.

I had chosen emergency medicine in part because, as a student, I was told that shift work was conducive to having a family, unlike more demanding specialties, like surgery. I have to admit that because the shifts were scheduled at all different times in a twenty-four-hour day, once I had my children, life often felt hectic and chaotic. In academic medicine, you're not just dealing with clinical work, you have your administrative and teaching responsibilities too. There was never enough time to get everything done.

As I garnered more administrative and educational titles at NYU (ultrasound fellowship director, then ultrasound curriculum director), I was able to reduce my clinical hours. These roles gave me more flexibility to have somewhat regular work hours, so I could be more present for my family, but I also had more work to do overall because the additional roles required more of my time. In academics, you often must prove yourself or your worth without really receiving anything tangible in return, at least in the beginning.

As faculty, we were supposed to be content with working at a prestigious institution, regardless of the fact that we were barely staying afloat.

———

By the time Natasha graduated from NYU in 2016, she was more than ready to leave. She had matched into the pediatrics program at another academic medical center in New York City, a place where she felt she would be valued, appreciated, and supported. Most notably, she made the conscious decision that she would not lead any diversity initiatives during her residency.

"I think one of the biggest things I learned at NYU is that I have to put boundaries in place to protect myself," she later told me. "If it's not helping me or my patients anymore, I'm not going to do it." She had come to NYU to learn how to be a physician, but she had left with another lesson entirely: the importance of preserving her emotional, psychological, and physical well-being from the burden of institutional racism. Someone else would have to forge the diversity, equity, and inclusion path at Mount Sinai, the institution where she had matched for residency. It wasn't going to be Natasha. It had been a hard lesson for her to learn—and one that eventually I would learn personally before my time at NYU was over. Years later, when Natasha and I reconnected, she would remind me that I had been the first person ever to encourage her to see a therapist to help provide some form of psychological support during her challenging times at NYU. She expressed her profound gratitude because it was the first time in her life that she had sought such support, and it had helped her.

The following spring, seven years after I had arrived at NYU, the medical school leadership asked me to take on a new role. This was an administrative leadership role as the faculty director for recruitment, retention, and inclusion in the Office of Diversity Affairs. In the aftermath of Barack Obama's presidency and Donald Trump's election, the US public was having a wider national conversation about racism and sexism. It was the year of the Women's March. Protests were happening in Central Park about the statue of J. Marion Sims, the so-called father of gynecology, who advanced his research by performing painful and traumatic procedures on enslaved Black women without their consent and without anesthesia. Students were ever more vocal in their discontent about the ways that the medical school was upholding racist practices and policies within health care. If I took on this new leadership role, it would be a chance for me to shift the institution's culture toward one that was more equitable and inclusive, yet I hesitated before saying yes.

The prior associate dean of diversity, a Black person, had been unceremoniously run out of the Office of Diversity Affairs after an infamous town hall where medical school leadership became very upset about the questions posed to them by students about the school's racist incidents and lack of diversity. This dean ended up not only leaving her position in the Office of Diversity Affairs, but she left NYU entirely. I soon discovered that another Black faculty member was leaving the Office of Diversity—and also NYU—around the same time as the associate dean. He was the person I would be replacing, and I had to get the scoop from him.

I asked this colleague if he would speak to me before he left, so we met outside behind the medical center in order to have a private place to talk. The roar of the cars passing overhead on FDR Drive did a good job drowning out our conversation. We stood inches away from each other and spoke in low tones.

"What's going on?" I asked him, as I inched closer, both of us instinctively feeling that we needed to keep our meeting secret. "You need to tell me what I'm walking into."

My colleague shared his professional frustrations about being passed over for opportunities for advancement in his department. He simply did not feel supported as a faculty member and had found a better opportunity at another hospital in the NYC area. As he told me his story, I took deep breaths, a constriction forming in my chest, making me feel nauseated.

And yet I went ahead and said yes anyway. To this day, I question why. I think the answer lies in my sense of duty and my optimism. Like my mother, I felt obligated to the students to make things better. I wanted to be a part of fixing the problem. I wanted to be a force for positive change. I think this is probably how so many Black faculty have felt walking into predominantly white institutions like NYU. We know that the environment is going to be tough on us, even harmful, but we feel we can't give up. I don't know if it's resilience or just sheer will, but whatever it is, it started with our ancestors—who had to bear so much, but who never gave up—and was passed on from generation to generation, all the way down to us.

PART III

UNBOUND

ELEVEN

Truth to Power

E ver since I was a little girl playing with my mother's black medical bag, I knew that I wanted to be a physician. After she died, following in her footsteps became even more meaningful to me. I was convinced that by going through medical school, training, and ultimately practicing medicine, I could embody her legacy. Never in a million years did I think I would leave academic medicine or do anything else with my career. And yet within two years of taking on the new role in NYU's Office of Diversity Affairs, that sense of certainty was gone.

From the moment I accepted the new job, there were problems. In addition to my focus on recruitment and retention of Black faculty and other faculty of color, I was tasked with addressing gender disparities within the school. A faculty engagement survey had revealed, unsurprisingly, that women who were junior faculty felt that, compared with them, their male peers were receiving more mentorship, sponsorship, and promotions.

Concurrently, national studies were coming out citing *disturbingly* high rates of sexual harassment in medical school, with between 20 and 50 percent of women students reporting they had experienced harassment from faculty, staff, and even patients. I hadn't realized just how pervasive sexual harassment is until then. As a student at Harvard Medical School, I'd had two distinct interactions that left me rattled, but I had assumed they were isolated incidents. My classmates had never shared any concerning stories. The first time was when a white male patient declared, "Wow, you're hot," as I walked into his hospital room with my team. As if this weren't jarring enough, my senior resident and junior residents were all men—and none of them spoke up for me. I remember feeling overcome by a sensation of nausea and lightheadedness in the warm room as my eyeglasses fogged up. I felt paralyzed. After we left the room, not one of them acknowledged what had just happened. A few days later, I went to my clerkship director and reported what the patient had said and the lack of team response. My director ended up speaking to my entire team, and they all apologized to me, but I never felt safe with them after that. The second incident was with my site director for pediatrics. One evening when I was on call, we were sitting down discussing a patient case and he looked over at me and said, in a lighthearted way, "You're going to be a looker once you get your braces off and you get contact lenses." I was so shocked, I didn't respond. I remember acting like I didn't hear him and continuing to discuss the case. This time, I didn't speak up, I just tried my best to avoid being with my site director when I was alone. There was part of me that tried to rationalize his comment, saying he didn't mean any harm, but I soon came to the realization that what he had said was completely inappropriate.

I started my new diversity role at NYU in October 2017, the same month that the #MeToo hashtag caught fire on social media, launching a movement and a national reckoning around sexual harassment and violence against women. I admit that I felt internally conflicted about the #MeToo movement because it was clear to me that Black women had been erased, excluded. It felt like a movement led by and for white women. Even the phrase was misattributed to Alyssa Milano, when Tarana Burke had coined it and founded the movement in 2006. It felt like the only reason why sexual harassment was becoming a headline was because affluent white women were the survivors and speaking openly about it. The movement didn't feel intersectional to me. Despite my concerns, I felt galvanized, realizing this was a long-overdue moment to have a reckoning on gender inequities and sexism within my own institution.

I decided that as a first step, I would do something with largely symbolic value. I went ahead and created an e-newsletter recognizing the work and accomplishments of women faculty. This would go out to the whole NYU community. It wasn't anything groundbreaking, but I felt it was a start. I put together the content and got someone to help with the design, but when I submitted the newsletter to my leadership for the necessary approval, they shot me down. Their response floored me: "No, we cannot put out this newsletter—it's not inclusive of men." Apparently if we celebrated and highlighted women in the medical school, faculty who were men would feel left out.

Okay, I thought. If that idea was too threatening, then what would be acceptable? My next idea was to organize an all-women faculty meet and greet to help junior faculty meet senior faculty and perhaps spark a mentor-mentee relationship. This raised no objections. A few months later, to my surprise, I was given approval to organize a Grand Rounds event on dealing with racist patients. Ever since Trump's election in 2016, there had been a marked uptick in explicitly racist incidents within hospitals. Whereas in the past the racism we encountered from patients tended to be more covert, now they felt emboldened, asking outright, for example, to be treated by white physicians. This was a crucial issue that needed to be addressed with urgency.

The speaker I invited to talk was a Fordham law professor who had written a piece on this subject in *The New England Journal of Medicine*, the premier medical journal. She was the first speaker on the issue in NYU's history, and as a result, the event attracted the attention of the press. A reporter from *The Wall Street Journal* had taken a particular interest in the topic of dealing with racist patients and was eager to speak with me. At the time, my resident was a Persian American man who had experienced multiple episodes of discrimination by patients at NYU who had assumed he was Muslim. I suggested she speak to him too. Before we spoke with the reporter about the event, however, my resident and I had to go through a twenty-minute media-training phone call with one of NYU's media representatives. The rep grilled me, asking exactly how I was going to answer each question from the reporter—word for word. He suggested several times that I modify a comment or statement to put NYU in a positive light. When

I told him that I wanted to share my own experiences of dealing with racist patients, he tried to discourage me from doing so. In the end, the conversation left me shaken, and I knew that I would have to be careful when I spoke with the reporter. Fortunately, the event itself ended up being a huge success, with over three hundred people in attendance, and after the speaker's visit, NYU did work to put in place a policy for how to manage racist patients in the hospital setting (though the policy was not well publicized at all and few people actually knew about it). But my conversation with the media rep left me feeling that I was actively being muzzled.

Later that same year, I invited a different speaker to talk to faculty about gender equity. This speaker was well known and had published some excellent research about gender inequities and how women are less compensated and promoted less frequently in academic medicine. This time I was told that one of the deans would have to be on the pre-call to vet the speaker to make sure she wasn't going to say anything "too polarizing." The call was an extremely awkward experience. I listened, horrified, as my dean asked this highly accomplished academic to describe verbatim the research that she would be presenting during her talk and reminded her several times that she didn't want her to say anything too controversial or polarizing during the talk. My dean told her, "We want this to be a positive conversation. We don't want to make anyone look bad." I cringed. The speaker shared with me later that she had never been vetted in this way by an institution before and had found it humiliating.

To make matters worse, I had been given only a sliver of

protected time for my new role, a tiny amount compared with the work that needed to be done—which is often the case for diversity and anti-racism work. It just wasn't (and still isn't) valued by white institutional leadership. When I realized the protected time wasn't enough, I was forced to go back and forth between my chair and the medical school leadership to try to negotiate for more hours. I would dread meetings with my chair because each time I had to prove myself and my accomplishments; essentially, I felt like I was begging.

My chair was a middle-aged white man who, from the moment I first met him, made it clear he hadn't spent much time with Black folks and didn't know much about what diversity, equity, or inclusion work required. Our conversations always felt incredibly strained.

"Take a seat, Uché!" he'd exclaim as I walked into his spacious, well-furnished office. "How's everything going?"

"I'm fine," I'd reply as I tried to force out a genuine smile, my body tensing up, betraying my words.

We'd small-talk for the first few minutes. He'd always ask how Chris was doing because they had once met and bonded over baseball.

"How can I help you today?" he'd ask, knowing full well that every single faculty who walked into his office needed something from him, usually more protected time for our nonclinical obligations.

I'd come prepared, after having rehearsed the conversation out loud countless times.

"So . . . I'd like to share with you what I've been working on over the last few months," I'd begin nervously. Then I'd run down my list of projects and work, hoping he'd at least be somewhat impressed by what I had accomplished. By this time—the fall of 2017—I had developed a four-year integrated bedside ultrasound curriculum for the medical school, one of the first of its kind in US medical schools. I'd received a distinguished research grant from the medical school and had published about the curriculum in one of the top clinical ultrasound journals. The best part was that our students were giving the curriculum rave reviews. Not only did they love it, but they found it a helpful adjunct to learning about anatomy and pathophysiology. I was also doing most of the teaching and administrative work for the curriculum. In tandem, my colleague and I had started and developed our department's first emergency ultrasound fellowship, much like the one I had completed at St. Luke's Roosevelt. We usually had one to three fellows a year, and so by 2017 we had graduated about ten fellows. Our goal was to make them experts in the clinical use of emergency ultrasound and to support them in their research projects. Many of them went on to serve as ultrasound leaders in emergency medicine departments across the country. It was very time-consuming work, but I loved seeing their professional growth, and the time and effort felt worth it. Taking on the diversity work on top of my other duties had substantially increased my workload.

Eventually, after multiple meetings, my chair gave me an additional small amount of protected time for my diversity role, an amount that was still not anywhere near adequate. I knew NYU leadership had very limited understanding of or appreciation for the value and complexity of the work with which they had tasked me.

And that's when it hit me. The people in institutional power, mostly older white men, didn't really expect me to *do* anything in my new role. They wanted a figurehead; they didn't expect me to change anything. Maybe they thought I would just sit there quietly, making them look good. They didn't realize that I cared deeply about transforming the system, that this work had become my passion. Talking to my colleagues in other institutions, I learned that this wasn't just an NYU problem. It was an *academic medicine* problem. It was the same situation in medical institutions across the country. Almost every medical school has an office of diversity affairs, but most of them suffer from lack of staff or funding or institutional will or some combination of all three. This is the irony of the situation. We are placed in these roles presumably to effect change, but we are rarely given any formal training, as if our lived experience is enough. This is not to say our lived experience is not invaluable, because it is, but there are diversity, equity, and inclusion training programs out there that can be helpful for professional development in this space. I was never told, "Uché, this is your role, and we are going to invest in you and make sure you get the training and support that you need to be successful in your role." In some ways, that's the nature of academic medicine—you get thrown into positions and you either sink or swim, or you learn by doing. At the same time, it's hard to do substantive work or even have a positive outlook when you don't have the people, the resources, or the institutional support to effect real change.

When my former program director from residency found out about the diversity, equity, and inclusion work I was doing, he invited me to speak at an academic medical center in the South. I delivered two presentations to his department, one about gender equity and the other on unconscious bias. I loved developing the presentations and made sure to make them interactive. I always hated sitting in a lecture and having someone speak *at* me. Especially as I was dealing with issues of race and racism, I thought it was important to truly engage with the audience and get them out of their comfort zone. My presentations ended up being more like workshops than lectures.

I began with a few pictures of myself, talking about why I was called to the work. The first was a picture of my mother holding Oni and me at our baptism, followed by a picture of our dad, and a picture of our dad with us at our medical school graduation. The message I was trying to convey was that health equity work goes deep into my bloodline, that I was continuing my mother's legacy.

As I led the audience through the session, I asked them to share where they may have acquired their internal biases.

"My grandmother! She'd always speak poorly of Black people."

"School!"

"What about school?"

"Our textbooks. They were one-sided. They never told the full story, but I was too young to question it."

"The local news!"

And so on. During these brief interactions, I tried to facilitate as much soul-searching as possible. It was only the beginning of the journey for them and it wasn't anywhere close to a holistic solution, but I always felt that having courageous conversations like these at least helped in some way to get us closer to justice. Word got out that I could speak to diversity, equity, and inclusion issues, and I had begun traveling around the country regularly, invited by other medical institutions to give talks.

When I was working on these issues, I came alive. I felt filled with purpose. The work was so needed and there was clearly a demand. A year into my position in the Office of Diversity Affairs at NYU, however, I was feeling less supported in the role than ever. Every newsletter that the office published had to be vetted by the senior deans (older white men) for inflammatory content. Certain content deemed too inflammatory by their estimation was censored. We were discouraged from speaking about current events relating to racism with our Black students because, we were told, our job was to pacify them and not rile them up or groom them to become activists. When people would reach out for help dealing with situations of inequity and discrimination within their departments, I would have to tell them, "I'm sorry, I can't help because I'm not empowered to do so." It was incredibly disappointing. Even though I had seen people leave the Office of Diversity Affairs before me, I had somehow remained hopeful that I could make a real impact. What would a real impact have looked like? If NYU truly wanted to make a difference, they would have to become more intentional about hiring, developing, and promoting Black faculty and recruiting and retaining Black students, explicitly use a racial equity lens in running the organization, create space for conversations about racism, and acknowledge the institutional and systemic factors that prevent Black faculty, staff, and students from flourishing. But after trying and failing to even begin the *conversation* about racism at NYU, I decided the best way for me to continue in the job was to hover under the radar. I was going to focus on our medical students and work with the student diversity groups to be where I was needed most. But I was not going to push for more. I wasn't going to be able to show up authentically as a Black woman physician at work. It just wasn't possible.

In October 2018, it was finally time for me to go up for promotion from assistant to associate professor. I had been told by members of the promotion committee that it was going to be a slam dunk. My department had voted unanimously for me to go up for promotion based on my academic work in ultrasound education, at the time considered to be quite innovative. As a result, I was assumed to be a shoo-in. The day I was due to hear the results—the decision of the committee—I got a call on my cell phone from my chair.

"Uché," he said, "I'm really confused. You didn't get the promotion."

I felt like my heart had stopped. A feeling of nausea came over me. What had happened? I had been told that I'd more than met the criteria: a certain number of publications, mentoring, curriculum that I'd developed, leadership roles. But for some reason my work had not been appreciated. Even my chair was surprised, but I later found out that he didn't understand why I was so upset. I had spent hours upon hours developing a new ultrasound curriculum in the medical school and starting an ultrasound fellowship in my department. None of this had been considered academically rigorous enough for the purposes of promotion. The experience was a wake-up call that I and my work were neither appreciated nor valued at NYU.

Thankfully, there were other people in powerful positions at NYU who went to bat for me when my promotion was denied. They helped me to refine my promotion packet in a way that showed how powerful the work was and how highly the students rated my course, and four months later, in February 2019, my promotion was finally approved. Even so, the whole experience left me disillusioned, but also gave me clarity. I realized if I really wanted to address racial health inequities and systemic racism, I needed to be free to say and think what I knew to be true. If I couldn't do this work boldly and honestly at NYU, then I would have to do it from the outside.

I had been thinking for a while that I might want to start my own company to train clinicians and others involved in health care about racial health inequities and systemic racism. In other words, I would be addressing all the gaps in knowledge I had been seeing my entire medical career. I would be doing something to fix not just the symptoms, but the roots of the problem. I called my new venture Advancing Health Equity. In March 2019, I formed an LLC and developed a website offering keynote talks and trainings on bias, systemic racism, and racial health inequities. My intention was to do this work part-time while still holding down my position at NYU. The mission of the organization was to engage with health-care organizations to create more diverse, inclusive, and anti-racist workplaces with the end goal to provide racially competent care to Black patients. I would finally be able to do the critical work that I had always wanted to do, but now I could do it on my own terms.

During this period, my husband, Chris, and I were really struggling at home. Of course, any marriage is challenging when both parents have busy full-time careers and the children are very young, as ours were. By all appearances, we were a beautiful family. But the truth was, our marriage had become full of tension. As my focus on my diversity, equity, and inclusion work grew, Chris and I grew further apart. Both of our children were finally growing out of the baby phase. I was beginning to see my life and my purpose more clearly, as well as the choices I had made personally and professionally. My travel and increasing passion for equity work put a strain on our marriage. Eventually, Chris and I became like strangers living together, barely speaking to each other. Over time, I stopped sharing the exciting developments in my career outside NYU, as well as the difficult time I was having at work. We were no longer connecting. Other deeply painful conflicts and disagreements arose between us. We briefly tried counseling, but it only made our differences more obvious.

The situation at work was becoming equally unsustainable. In May, three months after I got my promotion, a colleague I had become close to called me into their office.

"Uché," they told me, "I need to share something with you."

They explained that there was an issue.

"Apparently, there's a Twitter thread that you were involved in and it's causing some consternation."

They showed me the thread. I recognized it immediately. It had all started with a tweet from the former dean of Harvard Medical School, my alma mater. He had tweeted in April of that year about portraits of white male scientists that had been taken down at the Brigham and Women's Hospital, where he was now on the faculty.

> When I last lectured in @BrighamWomens Bornstein auditorium, walls were adorned with portraits of prior luminaries of medicine & surgery. Connecting to a glorious past. Now all gone. Hope everyone is happy. I'm not. (Neither were those I asked–afraid to say openly). Sad.

When I'd read the tweet, I'd been appalled that someone with his status had made such an ill-informed comment. And so I posted a series of tweets in response:

> My twin sister and I are HMS alums. When I read your tweet this morning, I had a visceral reaction. Do you realize that the wall of "prior luminaries of medicine & surgery" also represents a wall of racist and sexist practices and policies?
>
> Do you realize there are many people who would have been on that wall but were not allowed into medical school? . . . Please learn the history. The wall represented racism, white privilege, white supremacy and sexism.

I felt I had been thoughtful about what I had written. Certainly, everything I had said was factually correct. But someone had forwarded the thread to leadership, who had decided my comments were "inappropriate." My colleague wouldn't tell me all the details, but they explained that the powers that be were very upset. In addition to the tweets, they weren't pleased to hear I'd gotten involved with Time's Up Healthcare, a wing of the larger Time's Up organization, which had been founded to advocate against gender inequity and sexual harassment in health care. They felt I was too political.

University of Georgia professor Dr. Kecia Thomas has actually written about this workplace phenomenon, which she describes as "pet to threat," in which those in leadership turn against their Black women employees. In her study, Thomas and her colleagues learned that Black women coming into predominantly white institutions are often made into a "pet" early in their careers. They are encouraged, mentored, and supported. But as they begin to gain confidence in their jobs, these same women start to encounter hostility. Suddenly, they are perceived as a threat. They begin to be excluded from meetings and conversations. They start to feel isolated and alienated. An institution that was once welcoming becomes a place of marginalization. That was exactly my experience at NYU.

I started having trouble sleeping, trouble concentrating. I lost a lot of weight. I barely recognized myself in pictures. I doubted myself. I was angry with my leadership at work for not supporting me, angry with my husband because it felt like he wasn't understanding me as I tried to shed this old version of myself so I could grow into a new phase of my life. But as a Black woman, I didn't have the freedom to be angry. I didn't feel safe showing my anger, especially at work.

That July I had a second talk with my colleague about the Twitter thread.

"Leadership is still talking about it," they told me. "It's still an issue."

Then they said the words that changed everything for me.

"Uché, I'm telling you this as a friend," my colleague said. "I think you're going to have to find somewhere else to work."

I didn't ask them what they meant by that. Were they saying that I would have to leave because they were going to demote me, or they were going to make my life so miserable that I should get away for self-preservation? I was too scared to ask—and too scared to find out the answer.

I was already feeling exhausted and frustrated by the job. I knew I had to move on. But I had bills to pay. If I left NYU, where was I going to go? Did I even want to work in academic medicine anymore? It was becoming obvious to me that for my well-being, staying in this environment was not a healthy choice.

One day, not long after my colleague had called me into their office the second time, I was sitting at my desk and feeling totally dejected. I knew that the longer I stayed at NYU, the more I would feel like I was letting our students and patients down. But I was stalling. I had worked so hard to get to this point. My entire career had been built on the idea that I would establish a reputation for myself in academic medicine. So much of my identity was wrapped up in my affiliation with this prestigious organization. No one I knew just left academic medicine. Even within oppressive environments, we Black folks so often stick it out, doing our best to make a difference or because we need financial stability, or in elusive hopes that leadership will make changes.

I decided to pick up my phone and call my colleague Dara. The two of us had known each other since I was an intern at Kings County, and we had grown closer since we'd both ended up in positions at NYU. Unlike most of my close girlfriends, Dara was white. To this day, she remains the only white woman who I've had frank and candid conversations with about race and racism. She had also started her own company, which she ran part-time. I knew she would give it to me straight. Dara listened as I told her how worn down I was trying to effect change in an institution that was intent on preserving the status quo. Then she encouraged me to follow my heart.

"You don't have to stay at NYU," she said. "NYU doesn't define you. You can do anything. Just leave."

Dara's words released something in me. I realized she was right. Maybe I could leave academia and find an even greater fulfillment. I had spent most of my adult life checking off boxes: Go to college. Be premed. Attend medical school. Get a residency, a fellowship. Find a faculty position. Meet someone. Get married. Have kids. Live happily ever after. The end. For women, especially Black women, we are rarely granted the space to deviate from expectations—those of our loved ones, society, and everyone else in between.

I had tried to make it all work. But now I needed to do things my way.

Oni had always been my strongest source of support after our mother died. We had put considerable pressure on each other while grieving, but we remained incredibly close. We understood each other's pain. We understood each other's irreplaceable loss.

One day, we were on the phone talking about how sad and frustrated I was at NYU. Oni had been through her own ups and downs in her professional life. While at Montefiore Hospital, she had successfully applied for several large federally funded grants for her research. However, over time, she became frustrated by the slow pace of research and yearned for a way to make a larger-scale impact. After five years at Montefiore hospital, an opportunity presented itself in the role of assistant commissioner for the Bureau of HIV at the NYC Department of Health. It was a prestigious role. She took it. She had a national platform at the premier public health department in the country and had gone from leading a team of two people at Montefiore to leading a department of more than three hundred people with a $100 million budget. But the role came with challenges. It was hard being one of only a few Black women in leadership there. It was lonely. Like me, she was not fully able to inhabit her role as assistant commissioner because her voice was stifled by white men in positions of more influence than hers. At the same time, she was receiving constant messages that "You don't need to be here to make meaningful change."

"What do you think Mommy would say to me if she was still here?" I asked Oni.

"She would take your hands, pull you close to her, and say, 'I didn't raise you, put all this work into you, for you to feel unhappy and unsafe at work. You can do anything. Sky's the limit.'"

I sobbed into the phone as Oni uttered those words.

"You're right . . . you're right!"

I knew it was true. My mother would have been livid at how I was being treated. She had invested her precious time, energy, and love into us so we could have the choices that she never had. Oni reminded me that late in her career, our mother had quit her own position at Kings County because of limited opportunities for career growth, deciding to become board certified in geriatrics and taking on the role as a medical director at a nursing home in Manhattan. She had left because she wanted more. Now I wanted more too.

After the call with Dara and the conversation with Oni, I set wheels in motion. I developed a plan so that I could leave NYU but still support my family while I built my new business. I would get a job at an urgent care center part-time so that I could continue my clinical work without having to deal with working within a toxic institution. And this would give me time and energy to focus on my company, Advancing Health Equity.

Then I emailed my letter of resignation to my chair. As I clicked send, it was as if I could finally breathe again. It wasn't just that I was shaking off a job that was making me unhappy. I was also shaking off the weight of expectations: personal, parental, societal. I was done with being boxed in. I was going to do things my way.

That same summer in 2019, I gained the strength to tell Chris that I wanted a divorce. It was one of the most painful conversations I've ever had. There had been so many times before that day I'd wanted to bring up the prospect of a divorce with him, but I was scared of hurting him. I was scared to admit that our marriage was over. But I knew that staying for the wrong reasons would only hurt our family, especially our children, in the long run. As a child, I used to wake up to my parents' arguments. I didn't want the same for our children. I also knew that I had to be true to myself. Of course, the aftermath was not pretty. We would stay living in the same apartment for the next year while we went through the mediation process. It was hard. Really hard. There were many dark days. I would often call my sister crying.

And as always, Oni would remind me in her soothing, supportive voice, "Uché, this is just temporary. You will get through this."

My marriage was ending and so was my career in academic medicine. A lot of people, including members of my own family, thought that I didn't know what I was doing. When I told my father I was leaving my job, he immediately asked, seeming deeply concerned, "So what are you going to do now?" Sometimes I couldn't believe I was taking the leap either—giving up a role at a world-renowned medical institution where I had been successful by all objective measures, where I had a great salary, benefits, and job security, while at the same time divorcing my then-husband. I was effectively taking a huge demotion. To go from high-brow academia to a neighborhood urgent care center was considered by many a massive step down. But I knew if I stayed in the job and the marriage, I would be miserable, that I also worried about the toll it would ultimately take on my overall well-being. I left for myself.

My last day at NYU was in December 2019. After I finished my clinical shift, I went out the back of the building, quietly acknowledging to myself that this was the last time I would walk through these doors as a physician. Although I felt horrible about leaving my students to fend for themselves—I still feel terribly guilty about that—I hoped I could show them that they too could make nontraditional choices that felt right to them, that weren't always predetermined by others. I walked out that door feeling unencumbered, free, light, moving eagerly on to the next phase of my journey.

I made the decision that I would not go silently. I knew as soon as I wrote my letter of resignation that I wanted to go public about my experience at NYU, because I also knew it wasn't just NYU that was the problem. This was a widespread organizational and institutional problem, because systemic racism impacts every single social institution in this country, including medicine and health care. In January 2020, I published an opinion piece on *STAT*, a news website, titled "Why Black Doctors Like Me Are Leaving Faculty Positions in Academic Medical Centers." In the piece, I spoke openly about my experiences at NYU, about walking into an environment where Black people and other marginalized groups feel excluded, underappreciated, undervalued, only to have our concerns minimized when we try to address these issues with our superiors. Many people advised against writing the article, but I wrote it not only for myself, but for all others in my situation who might not have the same platform or influence that I did.

By that time, I had a sizable social media following on Twitter. I posted the article early the morning it came out, feeling a wave of relief initially, then fear. The next time I looked at my phone, the article had already been liked and retweeted hundreds, then thousands of times. Within twenty-four hours of *STAT* posting that article, I'd gotten so many nasty emails that I had to ask the editor to remove my contact details from the article. He said, "Of course I will. But I must tell you I've never had to remove an email from someone's first opinion piece." This blew my mind. I had gone through this toxic experience at NYU, and I had spoken up about it—and now I was experiencing hate-filled backlash. But for every negative comment there would be five more positive ones, telling me that my experience had been their own. I felt affirmed and validated.

By the end of the day, I received a slew of texts, emails, and phone calls from across the country, many from my Black friends and colleagues, but some from strangers who had contacted me through social media.

"Thank you, sis! You said what I couldn't say."

"We appreciate you speaking up for us."

"I couldn't have written it any better. You read my mind."

"Your essay resonated with me. I cried when I read it. I felt your pain and disappointment. I'm so sorry."

"I'm not even in medicine, but I relate to what you wrote. Thank you for affirming me!"

I noticed that very few of my white and non-Black colleagues from NYU reached out with words of support. Their silence was deafening—I will never, ever forget or forgive it. Even my original chair, who had stayed on as a faculty member, an amiable, progressive-minded older white man, someone I had grown close to during my time at NYU, never reached out to me. It felt like they all had decided together to align with a powerful institution instead of me, even though they had known me and worked closely with me for almost a decade. It felt like a gut punch.

Leaving academia was a fork in the road that I never could have seen coming. I was giving up the job security and prestige of working for one of the most revered academic medical institutions in the country. But I was exchanging it for something more precious to me: my freedom to speak truth to power. This was a new experience for me. For the first time in my professional life, I felt unbound.

After the *STAT* article was published, I imagined I would spend the rest of 2020 quietly and slowly building up my company. Things didn't work out quite the way I had planned.

TWELVE

All the Patients Look Like Us

I had left the superficial prestige of academia behind to take what most of my colleagues would consider a giant step down— leaving an associate professor position to work as a physician in a community-based urgent care clinic. But from my first shift in my new job, I never had any inkling of regret about leaving NYU. It felt right.

The plan was to work part-time in urgent care until my company was fully up and running. And in the meantime, life felt simplified. For the first time in many years, I could walk to work. I was assigned to three local urgent care sites in Brooklyn, but the one where I spent the majority of my shifts was in Bed-Stuy, the neighborhood right next to where I'd grown up. My childhood home was a fifteen-minute walk south and my own home was twenty minutes north. The area had become gentrified lately, and so my patients were a mix of Black folks who had been in the neighborhood for generations, newer residents who were mostly white millennials, and young families. Although the demographics had changed since my childhood, other than a few organic grocery stores and shiny new apartment buildings, physically Bed-Stuy looked very similar to how it did when I was younger. These were the same streets lined with historic brownstones of my youth, with a family-owned bodega or laundromat on every corner.

It felt like I was returning to my roots.

Urgent care clinics are small—really just a storefront with a small waiting area and about six exam rooms. The idea is to get people in and out as quickly as possible—and so most patients are seen within a few minutes. I was often the only clinician in the building, alongside a medical assistant and three scribes (who write up the charts for us and clean up the rooms). Like my mother had all those years ago at SUNY Downstate, I was caring for my neighbors. The difference was, unlike working in a teaching hospital, I was dealing with basic complaints: cold symptoms, people who had fallen and sprained a wrist or who needed routine vaccinations. It was all supposed to be incredibly manageable. Meanwhile, I was receiving a slow trickle of client inquiries for my company—to give racial and health equity trainings and keynote talks in various parts of the country, such as in New Hampshire at Dartmouth, and in Washington state from a large health-care system. I was learning how to be an entrepreneur, and my company kept me busy in the hours when I wasn't with patients or my kids.

Initially when I started my shifts in January 2020, we were in the midst of flu season and the center was quite busy. Then things slowed down in early February. It was like the calm before the storm. Of course, I had been hearing the news reports about COVID-19 in Wuhan, China, and as a physician I was aware of the threat it might pose if it came to the United States, but everything still felt far away. Then, at some point in February, a colleague at our care facility sent out a cheat sheet via a group chat. It was titled "What to Do if You Come in Contact with a COVID-19 Patient" and explained what to look for in terms of symptoms. I remember expanding the cheat sheet on my cell phone so I could see the fine print clearly. My heart sank as my eyes scanned the risk factors for those likely to develop severe COVID-19, including data from China about which patients were most susceptible: *elderly people; people with underlying medical problems such as diabetes, high blood pressure, asthma, obesity.* I thought about my father, who was in his late seventies. My heart continued to sink. *Diabetes, asthma, obesity. Underlying medical problems.* My heart sank even further. Due to structural inequities such as poverty, lack of access to care, and systemic racism, Black and Latinx communities carry a much higher chronic disease burden than whites. The thought occurred to me that if the virus came here, it was going to go straight to these communities—the ones that historically had been placed most at risk. I texted my sister the cheat sheet.

"Did you see this? I'm really worried."

Oni responded, "Yes, I saw. Not good. Not good at all."

I remember the very first week of March, a worried patient came in with mild cold symptoms, concerned that she had COVID-19. I told her to stay home until she felt better. Even if I had suspected she had COVID, I wouldn't have been able to say at that point because we didn't have any tests yet. I still couldn't conceive of what would become our reality less than ten days later when New York City was declared the epicenter of the pandemic in the United States.

By the time the governor and mayor locked down the city on March 20, 2020, an initial stream of COVID-19 cases had become a flood. Patient volume was surging at dramatic rates. As an emergency medicine physician, I always knew that in case of a disaster, I would have to be on call or available. It was like that after Hurricane Sandy in October 2012—much of the city was shut down but I still had to find a way to get to work and take care of our patients, even though very few patients arrived. This time, I knew that even though I was working in urgent care, it would probably be some of the busiest and most exhausting shifts I had ever experienced because of the volume of patients I would have to see. Thankfully, our urgent care leadership made sure that all staff had access to ample personal protective equipment (PPE). Eye covers were the only items in short supply, but masks, gowns, shoe covers, and gloves were readily available, and this gave me a layer of assurance because everything else was so unpredictable.

At first, we were seeing patients of different ages and backgrounds at our urgent care center. White, Black, Latinx people, the usual cross section of New Yorkers. And then suddenly, there was a shift. Almost overnight it wasn't the same racially and socioeconomically diverse population we had been seeing before.

Most of the staff working in our care center were Black and Latinx themselves—the front desk people, the manager, the scribes.

I remember turning to a young woman scribe named Alexis and saying, "This is strange, but do you notice that all the patients look like us now?"

And she replied, "Yeah, I do...."

Most of my patients were essential and service workers, many with underlying medical problems, people who couldn't do their jobs remotely, and people who were forced to take public transportation or who lived in crowded multigenerational housing. In other words, my patients were now overwhelmingly Black and Latinx New Yorkers.

My observation was soon supported by data showing that white affluent New Yorkers had disproportionately fled the city in those early months of the pandemic. Many went to second homes in Upstate New York, New Jersey, Connecticut, or Long Island, and some even moved out of the Northeast, which became stigmatized as the country's pandemic epicenter. Apparently, income became one of the strongest predictors of whether you stayed in New York City at the beginning of the pandemic or left. To me, it felt as if those white New Yorkers who left had essentially abandoned Black and Latinx New Yorkers to die. It was obvious that there wasn't going to be a collective response against this raging virus. It was every person for themselves.

I recall one day in the Prospect Park South area of Brooklyn in April 2020 when I was the sole clinician for a twelve-hour shift. I must have seen about a hundred patients during that span of time, the majority with COVID symptoms, the majority of them Black. The support staff and I called them "the walking wounded" because although most were sick, they were thankfully still able to walk in. I kept looking up at the computer screen and seeing the list of names grow longer, and when I glanced out the window, the line went all the way around the corner. I had been conditioned through my medical training to tough it out—and as I was new in the job at urgent care, I didn't want to give anyone any doubts that I couldn't do my job—but even so, I kept hoping that my supervisors, who always kept tabs remotely on patient flow, would send another colleague to help out. I kept wishing for the phone to ring and someone to say, "Uché, we're sending someone over to assist you!" Help never came.

We'd received tests, but only enough for two patients to test per shift. From a hundred patients, I had to choose only two whom I could test. It felt like an impossible task, but it had gotten to the point where if someone was symptomatic, I could diagnose COVID using their symptoms because everyone had the same story: "Oh, I have a little bit of fever, my head hurts, I'm feeling chest tightness and having trouble breathing." (At the time, we didn't know that about 30 percent of people with the virus do not even display symptoms.) The criteria for testing that had come down from the CDC was that we had to give priority to people who had recently traveled to one of the countries where COVID rates were the highest, like China, Italy, and Iran. In other words, right from onset, the testing criteria was biased against low-income New Yorkers—the working people who ended up contracting the virus even though they hadn't traveled. This is what happens when you don't see health care through an equity lens. The people you think about least are usually the ones most at risk.

I remember one patient in particular from that seemingly

endless day. She was an elderly Caribbean woman who came in assisted by a family member. Tall, about six feet, and rail thin, she could barely walk. After she struggled into the exam room, she slumped over into the chair, her body folding over on itself. Her breathing was rapid—about thirty breaths a minute, when normal range is about twelve to sixteen breaths a minute. Her eyes could barely open.

"Hello, ma'am . . . are you okay?" I asked as I bent down closer to examine her.

"I . . . feel . . . like . . . I'm . . . going . . . to . . . die." She was barely able to get the words out.

Although there were about thirty patients waiting to be seen at the time, I knew she was my sickest and I had to take my time with her. I held her hand tightly in my gloved hand and whispered to her, "Don't be scared. I'm going to take care of you."

I was able to get most of the history from her family member. She had developed a cough and fatigue the previous day, then a fever that reached 102 degrees that morning, and she had progressively become weaker. I tested her oxygen level. It was 78 percent. Normal is above 92 percent. We put a non-rebreather mask connected to an oxygen tank on her while the medical assistant called 911. We were able to get a quick portable chest X-ray that showed the hallmark COVID double-sided pneumonia pattern. I gave her Tylenol for her fever. EMS was there in less than ten minutes. The EMS workers lifted her onto the stretcher, strapped her in. I gave them a quick history and she was whisked away. I don't know what happened to her, but she stands out from the other patients I saw that day because she was so gravely ill.

We were barely two weeks into stay-at-home orders. At that point, we didn't even have preliminary data on the racial and ethnic demographic breakdown of the COVID-19 cases: who was being hospitalized and who was dying. Very few people were talking in the mainstream media about race and COVID-19, even those who spent their careers researching health inequities. We were all too shell-shocked by what was happening. I didn't know whether what I was seeing with the racial makeup of patient demographics at the urgent care was an NYC phenomenon or beyond, because the media wasn't reporting on COVID racial health inequities yet, but I knew I had to speak up about what I was seeing.

I decided to write an op-ed. I described what I was observing at work, my concerns that we would ultimately see this same pattern play out across the country. I submitted what I had written to *Slate*. An editor emailed right back and asked if they could interview me. The article, written by staff writer Julia Craven, was aptly titled "How Racial Health Disparities Will Play Out in the Pandemic: Dr. Uché Blackstock Explains How the Coronavirus Will Affect Black Patients, and Why That Terrifies Her." It was shared thousands of times over social media. It became one of the very first pieces to address racial health inequities in the pandemic. At the end of the interview, Julia asked me what was at stake with this virus. I answered, "Humanity."

I also told her that I was scared.

All of my speaking engagements and trainings for AHE had to be canceled because they were supposed to be in person, and we hadn't shifted to providing virtual services yet. I was asked to pick up more shifts at the urgent care center, and I started working three twelve-hour shifts a week, while responding to increasing requests to speak to the press. As the data started coming out, showing the surging numbers of Black people and other people of color contracting and dying from the disease, I felt further compelled to communicate the urgency of the situation and my observations. I made appearances on radio and TV, gave interviews for newspapers and magazines.

I soon became accustomed to going to work in my PPE—face mask, face shield, gown, shoe covers, and my hair in a cap. While I often worried about eventually running out of PPE, especially knowing what was happening at other NYC hospitals, it never happened. I was immensely grateful that there was one less thing to have to worry about. Even though I had spent my career in the unpredictable and chaotic emergency room setting, this was the first time I had felt fearful going to work. There was this constant sense of anxiety that a patient with COVID was going to walk through the door, that I was going to get sick, and that I would bring the virus home to my family. Sometimes I would walk into an exam room with a patient, breathe in the stagnant air, and wonder, "Is this going to be the time I get infected?" In those early days, there were so many unknowns about COVID. Sometimes, I would be scared even to stay in a room too long with a symptomatic patient. Initially, we were fully covered from head to toe in PPE because there was much we didn't know about COVID. As the weeks turned into months, masks and eyewear became most important as we learned that the virus was airborne. As soon as I walked in the door of my apartment at the end of my day, I took off my clothing and put it in a garbage bag. I felt contaminated, making sure to shower before hugging or kissing my kids.

Then there was the additional stress of our boys being home doing remote learning. Chris and I would trade off helping them with their schoolwork—and we also had a wonderful caregiver, Tata—but it was obvious that a three- and five-year-old could learn only so much online. They were full of energy. They would start jumping onto the furniture, bouncing off the walls. They ended up breaking numerous objects in our apartment because they would start fighting with each other because we couldn't go out and there was not enough to do. It felt like everything was breaking apart all around me.

Chris and I had both decided finally to move forward with divorce proceedings. I had suggested mediation, as I thought it was the least antagonistic way to proceed and would keep the boys our main priority. He had agreed. There was so much tension in the apartment at the time. My only escape was to go to work. But work was hell. As I walked there each day, the streets of Brooklyn—usually so busy and full of people at all times of the day and night—were eerily quiet. The subways were virtually empty. Stores were either closed or deserted. It was like walking through a ghost town. As these were the only moments I had to myself, I actually savored them.

One patient stays in my mind from that spring. He was an older Black gentleman who came in by himself sometime in May; he had fallen at home and he didn't look good. I checked his vital signs, and they were very concerning: his oxygen level was 80 percent and he had a fever, high heart rate, and shortness of breath. I could hear him wheezing every time he took a deep breath. Even without testing him, I knew he had COVID. We did a chest X-ray, which showed the double-sided pneumonia. There was no way this man should go home.

"I'm going to call an ambulance, you need to go to the ER," I told him.

He shook his head no. "I'm not going," he said.

"Why not?" I asked.

"I don't trust hospitals. I'm safer at home."

This man had heard the news reports that the ERs were overrun, that there weren't enough beds and staff for COVID patients. He wasn't the only one who decided it would be safer to visit an urgent care center. New Yorkers came by the thousands and tens of thousands to urgent care sites all across the city, including ours, because ERs were beyond capacity. As a result, there would always be at least a few very sick patients per shift who walked in with shortness of breath and oxygen levels in the low sixties, numbers that were incompatible with life. Very few of these patients wanted to go to the ER, mistakenly believing that we were equipped to care for critically ill patients at urgent care. We were not. What these patients did not understand was that we did not have the airway equipment that would allow us to put in a breathing tube to help people breathe. We also didn't have a wide supply of intravenous antibiotics or medications needed for extremely sick people. Often I was the only health-care professional at a site, so we didn't have an extra set of trained hands to help, and there was nowhere to admit the patient because we were not a hospital. That day, I had a long conversation with my elderly patient, trying to persuade him to change his mind and go to the hospital. I explained how sick he was and the kind of treatment and care he needed. He told me he was also concerned that his insurance wouldn't cover the whole cost of his stay and that he wouldn't be able to afford the medical bills. If I wouldn't treat him, then he was going to go home. This elderly man had come to urgent care by himself; there was no one else to whom I could appeal. He simply refused to let me call the ambulance. Instead, he took his walker and shuffled out the door. I watched him go with a very heavy heart—before moving on to the next patient, and the next one. In the coming days, our follow-up service called him but I never found out what happened, if he recovered or not. To this day, I am fearful he didn't survive, like so many New Yorkers who stayed home rather than risk going to the hospital in those early days.

The pandemic was making it abundantly clear that structural racism was and is a key driving factor of the social determinants of health. Lack of adequate health insurance and, understandably, lack of trust in the medical system were contributing factors to who lived and who died. People who had jobs that were putting them on the front lines were at far greater risk of being exposed to the virus. People living in overcrowded housing—which is more likely to occur in our communities because of lack of affordable housing and systematic exclusion from home ownership opportunities—were also more likely to be infected. Even thinking about who is using public transportation and who is less likely to be able to afford a car, we're looking at our communities.

In the first half of 2020, Black Americans' life expectancy declined almost three years to an average of seventy-two years, compared with a loss of almost one year for white Americans (now seventy-eight years). Meanwhile, Black Americans not only were twice as likely to die of COVID as white Americans but were also dying at rates similar to those of white Americans who were ten years older. Moreover, racial inequities were most striking at younger ages; for example, Black people ages forty-five to fifty-four were seven times more likely to die of COVID than similarly aged white Americans.

In June 2020, I was asked to become a medical contributor at *Yahoo! News*, speaking on news events related to racial health inequities. I saw my media work as a form of advocacy. I felt a near desperate urgency to share my thoughts—and people seemed to need the information and insight I could offer them. I used this new platform to explain the many ways that systemic racism has limited the opportunities and resources that Black Americans have, and how it had placed us in a situation in which we were among the most vulnerable to this virus. The pandemic was showing us how deeply embedded racism is in this country, in every aspect of the lives that we lead, and I was speaking out about it.

No longer muzzled by my role at NYU, I could say what I wanted to say. In the midst of the crisis, I found my voice.

THIRTEEN

Where I'm Supposed to Be

Without planning it, I had left academic medicine to build a reputation as a health equity advocate at a pivotal moment in US history. On March 13, 2020, twenty-six-year-old Breonna Taylor, an emergency medical technician in Louisville, Kentucky, was sleeping in her bed when she was shot eight times. Her murderers were members of the Louisville Metro Police Department who used a no-knock warrant to invade her home looking for drugs that were not there. By the end of May, her boyfriend's distressed call from the night of her shooting had been released, bringing her story to national attention. Just a few weeks before Taylor's murder, twenty-five-year-old Ahmaud Arbery, who was out jogging, was shot in cold blood by armed white vigilantes in Glynn County, Georgia. On May 5, video of that footage was released to national outcry. Then, on May 25, forty-six-year-old George Floyd was murdered by a white Minneapolis police officer who used his knee on Mr. Floyd's neck to pin him to the ground for eight minutes and forty-six seconds, while he begged for his life, pleading with the cops to let him breathe. A teenage girl, Darnella Frazier, somehow found the courage to videotape the event. Two days after that, Tony McDade, a thirty-eight-year-old transgender man, was shot and murdered by a police officer in Tallahassee, Florida. These events, happening in such rapid succession, during a pandemic that was disproportionately taking the lives of Black people, sparked over one hundred days and nights of marches and protests throughout the US.

At the urgent care centers where I worked during that summer, we experienced a period of respite from the high number of COVID cases, our patient volume steeply decreasing. Often while on shift, we'd hear shouting from outside: "Black Lives Matter! Black Lives Matter!" On any given day, three to four protests would pass by, and if there were no patients waiting to be seen, I'd go outside with our staff, wearing our scrubs and shouting in unison with the protesters, pumping our fists and yelling, "Black Lives Matter!"

Every time, I'd wish I was out there with them. When we were growing up, Oni and I had protested with our parents at the United Nations against apartheid in South Africa and in Bensonhurst and Howard Beach after local racist hate crimes involving Black male victims. One weekend that summer of 2020, following our parents' lead, Oni and I took our boys to Times Square for a large protest sponsored by several physician groups. "Mama, where are we going?" my older child asked. I explained to him what had happened to George Floyd and Breonna Taylor and that we were going to demand justice for them and their families. I couldn't tell if my three-year-old and five-year-old were more in awe of being in Times Square with its tall buildings and gaudy signs or if they could feel the energy of the moment.

After a few initial words by organizers, we started walking as a group through Midtown with our signs. "No Justice, No Peace!" we chanted. My older child held my hand tightly as we rounded the corner from Broadway onto Forty-Second Street. "Mama, tell me more about Breonna," he said.

I explained that she was an ER technician, that she had wanted to help people, that she was someone's daughter, someone's sister, that she was loved. I told him that I was angry. I explained that we Black folks had been crying out against police violence and murders since forever, but now Americans of all skin colors and walks of life were as outraged as we had been. That this outcry of anger and demand for change was long overdue.

To this day, I'm still furious—not only about cold-blooded killings such as George Floyd's, but that it took a Black man being violently murdered on video for white America to finally wake up. Would the awakening be temporary or permanent? Only time would tell. I'm an optimist by nature, but historical patterns and human nature teach me that the awakening was more likely to be fleeting. The immediate impact, however, was considerable. After Mr. Floyd's murder and news of the other recent murders of Black people became national news, more people felt galvanized to do something. As individuals posted Black squares on their Instagram pages to show solidarity with the Black Lives Matter movement, organizations and institutions appeared to be starting to get their act together in every industry and discipline, including medicine and health care. The connections were clear. Systemic racism in policing took Black people's lives and so did systemic racism in medicine and health care.

Black researchers and health-care professionals had been doing rigorous health equity research for decades, and I felt honored to communicate and amplify their important research to the media and public through TV appearances, op-eds, and social media. In June 2020, as a result of the visibility I'd gained due to my media appearances, I was invited to testify in front of the House Select Subcommittee on the Coronavirus Crisis for a hearing on racial health inequities. This was my opportunity to cogently present the case for how systemic racism had left Black communities and other communities of color more vulnerable to the detrimental impact of coronavirus. The hearings were taking place virtually, and so I gave my testimony on Zoom. My boys, who were learning remotely at home, were playing in the adjacent room. I remember feeling anxious excitement as House Majority Whip James Clyburn, who headed the committee, introduced me and I shared my prepared speech.

"Black men have the shortest life expectancy," I reminded the members. "Black babies—the highest infant mortality rate. Black women—the highest maternal mortality rate, and this trend persists despite socioeconomic status and level of formal education. Even the chronic stress of living with daily racism results in 'the weathering effect,' the premature physiologic aging of Black Americans' bodies.

"Living in this country has essentially made Black Americans sick. And over the last three months, we have witnessed a crisis layered upon another crisis as Black communities across this country have borne the greatest burden of illness and death from the novel coronavirus.

"More than one in two thousand Black Americans have died.... If Black Americans had died at the same rate as white Americans, about thirteen thousand Black Americans would still be alive today."

I spoke about the distrust among Black Americans toward the health-care system, reminding the legislators of its roots in a horrific legacy involving centuries of neglect, abuse, and exploitation of Black communities, layered under the many current-day inequities.

"Structural racism, through social and economic policies that disadvantage Black people, has placed Black Americans at risk for illness and death," I explained. "It has been the key driving force behind the factors that determine an individual's and communities' health outcomes."

I implored the committee to use this moment to act urgently and swiftly to mitigate these widespread and appalling racial health disparities, to address structural change in the form of safe and adequate housing, employment, access to quality education, access to healthy foods, and health care for all.

"This country desperately needs a truth and reconciliation process around the racist policies, economic systems, and institutions that have left Black lives devalued," I insisted. "This is an opportunity to explicitly acknowledge unjustified past and ongoing wrongs, engage with Black communities, and rebuild them equitably."

I appreciated the opportunity to advocate for health equity and to even educate some of the congresspeople who doubtlessly believed that there was something inherently deficient in Black people—and that's why we were being so negatively impacted. Only time would tell if they would listen and if words would turn into deeds.

When it comes to the Black health-care crisis, everything is intertwined; nothing happens in isolation. In the US, around one thousand people are shot by police officers every year. Black Americans are three times more likely than their white counterparts to die during a police encounter. Statistics from a 2018 National Academy of Sciences study show that one in one thousand Black men or boys will be killed by police. Yet recent research also shows that when communities have high rates of police brutality and negative interactions with the police, community members *also* have a distrust of health-care institutions. If you think about it, it makes sense that an interaction within one institution (the police force) could influence people's desire or feelings about another institution (their local hospital or health-care professionals). One study suggests that the greater police presence in Black versus white neighborhoods may contribute to the persistent disparity in preterm births between Black babies and white babies. Racism is not always as overt as it was in the killing of Mr. Floyd and so many others. So often it's covert, invisible to many, yet completely pervasive. You can count the number of Black people murdered by police, but how do you account for people who die because they're too scared to go for a regular health checkup?

With every news story of another instance of police homicide, my company, Advancing Health Equity, began to be inundated with requests from health-care organizations and institutions for remote health equity trainings, listening sessions, and organizational assessments. Everyone had different requests, but they were all connected to addressing racism. People were truly shaken by what had happened to Mr. Floyd and others, and they finally wanted to talk about how systemic racism impacted the health of Black people.

I made the trainings feel very personal. I shared my own story about how my parents had tried to get a mortgage in the 1970s, but due to the legacy of redlining they struggled to get one. I talked about my neighborhood in Brooklyn that had no grocery store when I was growing up, and how we had to go elsewhere to get fresh food. Other participants of color shared their own stories, saying they had grown up in underserved areas, but just blocks away there were well-resourced white neighborhoods. Many of the white participants had never thought about why that might be. They had just accepted that that was the status quo and didn't interrogate their own beliefs.

Many times, I was the only Black person in the Zoom room. Those conversations were often very challenging. There were a lot of uncomfortable silences.

"I'm nice to all of my patients," one white physician insisted. "I'm not sure what this has to do with me?"

Another physician questioned why I was telling the group about redlining, insisting that because his family had struggled to buy a house—but had finally managed it—Black families could too.

I took a deep breath. "This discussion today is just the beginning of a new journey for you," I replied firmly. "I know as physicians you think you're experts in caring for your patients, but there's a lot you've never learned in school, in training, or in practice, and those gaps in your education are leading you to harm your patients. That's why I'm here today. You can do better. You must do better. Your Black patients and patients of color are suffering and dying."

I continued, informing them about the complex history of oppression that got us to this point. I spoke about how for white people living in a society with systemic racism, internalized societal messaging shows up in the numerous studies that indicate that many white physicians and clinicians don't listen to Black patients. I connected the dots between how systemic racism also impacts housing, employment, education, access to health care, and access to healthy foods. I would often leave these trainings emotionally exhausted, having to ground myself and recover after each session. Even so, I knew it was worth it because of our patients, Black patients, who continue to drive me to do this work. It's not just a job for me, it's my purpose.

One of my earliest trainings was for Planned Parenthood of Greater New York, and it took place way upstate, in a part of New York that's not known for its progressive politics. I remember feeling a little more nervous than usual before the training began, wondering how what I had to say would be received. As I always did, I walked the participants through the stages of the training, explaining to them the ways in which systemic racism had led directly to our current Black health crisis, and the ways in which they, as health-care professionals, could be part of the solution.

There was one white woman physician who I noticed looked particularly withdrawn and disengaged that day. I worried I wasn't getting through to her. After the training, when I went to check my email, I was surprised to find I had a note from her.

"I was so overwhelmed during your session," she wrote. "It wasn't easy for me, but I feel awakened now. I really want to help. Please let me know what else I can do."

I had interpreted her reserved expression as a lack of engagement. In fact, she was absorbing the information and processing it—and had come away realizing that she could play a more active role. This was exactly the impact I had hoped the trainings *would* have. I wrote her back immediately, thanking her for her email and offering a series of follow-up calls to strategize what her next steps could be at her workplace. It was interactions like those that made me feel hopeful. I knew that we couldn't move or change every participant, but I knew there were some white participants who did want to do better and do the work to dismantle racism in their workplace. She would email me frequently with updates. "This is a marathon, not a sprint," I reminded her.

Although I started my company by offering talks and workshops to those in the medical realm, I soon added organizational assessments and equity audits—and brought in skilled facilitators to help run the trainings. During the assessments and audits, we would interview leadership and staff, facilitate focus groups with key constituent groups within the organization, and review organizational practices, procedures, and policies. Then we would summarize our findings, make recommendations, and lay out a plan for how to make these workplaces and organizations more racially equitable. We told our clients that change starts at home. If they wanted the health care they offered to be more racially equitable, they had to create equitable workplaces first.

There was so much work to do. The US is the wealthiest country in the world, yet we have the worst health outcomes out of any high-income country, and in part that's because our persistent racial health inequities are so profound. Any health-care organization that wants to address health inequity must recognize the root causes and identify strategies at multiple levels.

For so many white Americans, 2020 was a wake-up call. For Black folks, it was one of the most exhausting and devastating years in recent history. The pandemic rolled on, leaving hundreds of thousands of lives in its wake. In December 2020, we faced yet another tragedy, the death of Dr. Susan Moore, a Black woman physician from Indianapolis. While desperately ill in the hospital with COVID-19, Dr. Moore made a viral video from her bed, with an oxygen tube in her nose. Despite her compromised state, she still summoned the strength to post a video to Facebook about her mistreatment. She described how her white doctor "made me feel like I was a drug addict," refusing to prescribe her additional painkillers when she complained of pain—even though he knew she was a fellow physician. She related how he rejected her plea for additional doses of remdesivir; how "he did not even listen to my lungs; he didn't touch me in any way"; how he suggested she should just go home.

"This is how Black people get killed, when you send them home and they don't know how to fight for themselves," Moore said, struggling to speak.

Less than three weeks later, she was dead at age fifty-two. My first thought watching her video was "This could be me." My education, my socioeconomic status, even the fact that I was a physician—none of this was enough to protect me as a Black person in the US health-care system.

But there were other reasons why the distribution of lifesaving therapies for COVID-19 was significantly delayed for Black patients. Not only have white physicians like the one who treated Dr. Moore failed to listen to us, we also later learned that readings from pulse oximeters—which measure oxygen levels in the blood, and which were used throughout the pandemic to assess patients for severity—were inherently biased. Throughout the pandemic, low oxygen readings from pulse oximeters have been the gold standard for how physicians assess the need for more aggressive medical care in COVID-19 patients. The problem has been that these devices actually *overestimate* blood oxygen levels in patients with darker skin tones, making those patients seem healthier than they actually are. According to a recent study, readings taken from arterial blood samples found pulse oximeters were *three times less likely* to detect low oxygen levels in Black patients than they were in white patients. These inaccuracies persist across other racial groups, with Hispanic and Asian patients also affected.

UCHÉ BLACKSTOCK, MD

Undetected low oxygen levels have inevitably led to delays in patients of color receiving lifesaving COVID-19 therapies such as remdesivir and dexamethasone, or patients being sent home without any treatment at all.

Bias in pulse oximeter readings is something researchers have raised concerns about for decades. Yet because this information has never become part of the medical curricula, the vast majority of physicians—myself included—had no idea these devices were unreliable until two years into the pandemic. And even in the midst of a COVID-19 epidemic that killed over a million Americans, the medical establishment still couldn't find the will to replace these pulse oximeters with devices that would give accurate readings—not just for white patients but for all of us.

Throughout 2020 and into 2021, I continued to practice clinically in urgent care. Although we were no longer under a stay-at-home order, the crisis of the pandemic was far from over. In early 2021, after multiple appearances, I was invited to become a medical contributor exclusively for MSNBC. I would often be asked to speak on the intersection of health care and racism, which meant talking primarily about COVID-19 and its heavy toll on Black Americans. Change never happens overnight—and when it comes to racism in the United States, change moves at an infuriatingly glacial pace. But it can't happen if the rest of the public isn't aware of the necessity of change. If nothing else, unlike anything had in the past, the pandemic opened much of the public's eyes to systemic racism in health care.

FOURTEEN

A Better Way

Often, I would get stopped on the street by neighbors or people from my community who had seen me on TV, asking me for medical advice or sharing supportive words.

"Dr. Blackstock!" they'd call out.

Of course, whenever I heard those words, I immediately thought of my mother. She had been that person who everyone felt comfortable approaching in the street and asking for advice, recommendations, or referrals. She was always happy to lend people her time and share her expertise.

Now it was my turn. Many times, walking down the main drag in my neighborhood, someone would say, "Oh, doc, I saw you on TV, I need to ask you about something..."

In late 2020 and early 2021, when the first vaccines against COVID-19 became available, that was all anyone wanted to talk about.

At that time, I spoke frequently on TV and radio about the

vaccine rollout and the ways I could see that it was already excluding Black and Latinx communities. Access was an issue in the early days of the rollout because distribution was being done mainly from hospitals. Due to systemic racism, many Black communities don't have enough hospitals or clinics. Also, community members may avoid such institutions due to medical mistrust, or because immigration or insurance status is a concern. But there were other issues as well. In the beginning, because health-care workers and the elderly were prioritized for vaccines, it gave people the idea that there was a scarcity of vaccines, sending the wrong message that vaccination wasn't for everybody, just for special groups. While the COVID-19 vaccines were developed quickly, there wasn't enough emphasis put on educating and informing people about the fact that no steps had been skipped or missed in the development and testing of the vaccines, and that the vaccines were safe and effective as a result. Instead, we had vaccines that appeared to have been developed very quickly and were available only in hospitals and only to certain groups—so the message about vaccines gleaned by our communities was that they were being excluded, that "this isn't for you," and that the vaccines could be risky due to having been developed at such speed.

One day in December 2021, I was walking along the main drag in my neighborhood.

I heard, "Yo . . . Uché!"

I turned around and spotted my former barber, Gee, sitting in his car, waiting for the barbershop to open. Whenever I see him around, we chat, even though I don't need his services anymore since growing my hair into long locs.

Gee got out of his car and we met on the sidewalk. At over six feet tall, he hovered over me and had to bend down to give me one of his usual warm bear hugs.

After we hugged, he stepped back a little, looking down at me with a serious look on his face.

"Uché, I got questions," he said quietly, leaning in toward me.

"About what?"

"The vaccine. I don't have health insurance. I don't have a doctor," he continued. "You're the only doctor I know. The only one I trust."

We ended up arranging a call for a week later. I spoke with Gee and his adult daughter on the phone for almost an hour.

"How was the vaccine developed so quickly?" he asked. "How do I know it's safe? What about long-term complications?"

I could tell he had been thinking about and wrestling with these questions for a while. He even mentioned how the messaging from the CDC over the past year has been confusing for him. I told him he was not wrong about the confusing messaging, but that the vaccine was safe.

Three weeks after our conversation, Gee went and got his first dose of the COVID vaccine. He shared with me that what had helped change his mind was my reassurance that he didn't need insurance and that I had recently gotten my kids vaccinated.

I was touched that he had felt safe enough to share his questions, but it also saddened me to my core that he didn't have another health-care professional in his life whom he trusted. This is how fractured the relationship between Black communities and the US health-care system has become. We need a system where insurance isn't a barrier, where there are many more Black physicians and health-care professionals, and where there is greater access to quality care within our communities. We need a healthcare system that embraces people like my barber, that welcomes them.

We don't have that system. Instead, we have a decentralized, hybrid health insurance system that is mostly privatized, in which hospitals, insurance companies, and physicians seek to maximize profit. In 2018, about 55 percent of the US population was covered under employer-sponsored insurance. The remainder were covered under Medicaid, Medicare, and the Affordable Care Act. That still leaves about 10 percent of our population uninsured.

Black Americans were initially slow to sign up for the vaccine, and no wonder. Dating back to the days of slavery, Black people have been used as guinea pigs for medical advancements, including the development of vaccines. The very first vaccine in this country was actually introduced by an enslaved African known as Onesimus. Although we don't know Onesimus's true name or birth date, we do know he was enslaved to Cotton Mather, a Puritan minister, who renamed him, and that Onesimus's advice to Mather was instrumental in bringing inoculation to colonial America. The variolation method of vaccination, in which a small drop of a disease is introduced through punctured skin as a way of protecting people against infectious outbreaks, had long been practiced in Africa and sub-Saharan countries. Onesimus explained the principle of variolation to Mather, in which the immune system is triggered to make antibodies, and Mather became an advocate for the practice, enlisting a local doctor, Zabdiel Boylston, to test the theory. Boylston was intrigued, and began injecting smallpox lymph (the colorless liquid found within the smallpox vesicle) into enslaved people in his home. When a smallpox outbreak spread through Boston, killing hundreds of people, Mather became a staunch advocate for inoculation. His insistence that vaccines could protect against disease was met with widespread derision and suspicion, especially as he had turned to an enslaved man for medical advice.

By the time smallpox broke out again during the Civil War, however, the efficacy of vaccines in protecting against infectious diseases was more widely accepted. The problem was, there weren't enough vaccines available to inoculate soldiers, so army medics on both sides of the conflict deliberately infected enslaved babies and children in order to harvest vaccine matter from them. A Confederate doctor named James Bolton actually traveled around the state of Virginia injecting enslaved people, mainly children, with smallpox and then returning at a later date to see if their bodies had created the lymph needed for vaccination. On the other side of the conflict, a Union physician infected a group of formerly enslaved children in a refugee camp in Missouri with the virus, again to extract lymph from their bodies in order to vaccinate soldiers.

Such horrific historical abuses and traumas—alongside the more well-known atrocities of the US Public Health Service's Tuskegee Study of Untreated Syphilis in the Negro Male and the harvesting of Henrietta Lacks's cells without her consent or knowledge—are important contexts in understanding contemporary concerns about vaccines in Black communities, but they are not the main factor. The abuses aren't just historical. They're happening now. Every day in this country, Black people find themselves faced with a medical system that doesn't listen to us, doesn't value us, and often actively harms us. During the pandemic, we were left to suffer and often die. Such incessant assaults on our basic humanity have created an instinctive mistrust that is well-founded. Never at any point in our lives or the lives of our ancestors have we been well served by our health-care system. So why should we trust it now?

Anytime there is mistrust, misinformation has an opportunity to flourish. The vaccine was one of the most important ways we could protect our community, which had suffered so terribly and disproportionately during the pandemic. But the Biden-Harris administration found itself working against history to win trust, reflected in early vaccination rates, with Black people having the lowest proportion of vaccinations among any racial or ethnic group, even though we were almost three times as likely as our white counterparts to be hospitalized because of COVID-19, and twice as likely to die.

Oni joined me in writing op-eds about the vaccine rollout. After seeing me leave NYU to focus on my company and watching other friends start their own health equity consultancies, she had founded a consultancy of her own, Health Justice, in 2020. Together, we called for Black Americans to be prioritized for the vaccine, given the pandemic's disproportionate toll on Black communities. Something similar had already been done with Indigenous peoples in Australia and Canada. We felt that removing or lowering age cutoffs for Black Americans could go a long way toward increasing access to one of the most impacted communities while accounting for structural racism's toll on Black lives. We argued that systemic racism prematurely ages Black Americans and that vaccine age cutoffs early in the rollout had essentially discriminated against Black Americans, a demographic group that is more likely to have chronic diseases at younger ages.

We urged the Biden-Harris administration to act to ensure that Black Americans would not be left out of the rollout process. We explained the importance of meeting people where they were, in all senses of the expression. We needed to bring the vaccine to communities, to churches, libraries, and barbershops, and not just hospitals. And we needed to have a conversation around the vaccine, listening to people's concerns and working with that hesitancy, not against it, as I had done in conversation with my barber. The Department of Health and Human Services and the CDC needed to mandate that states collect complete racial and ethnic demographic data, including zip codes of those who were being vaccinated, to help target public health efforts toward Black communities. Because the local and state public health systems are so disconnected, that effort to have complete data has never been fully realized.

Above all, we called for a collective, holistic response to this crisis, not one that placed such a large emphasis on individuals to protect themselves with a vaccine. People in our communities were more at risk because they didn't have sick leave or they didn't have health insurance, or because they were working in environments that put them at high risk of being exposed, or because they had to take public transportation, or because they were often in multigenerational living situations that put them at further risk, or all of the above. These are the fundamental factors we need to address going forward to protect our communities, factors that go far beyond a shot in the arm.

The pandemic was a spotlight revealing the kind of structural violence that usually doesn't get airtime on national TV. But we were also getting a glimpse of a better way.

On one of my shifts at the urgent care clinic, I remember being called to the front desk to see a patient who had come in while on his food delivery shift. He still had on his orange vest and his helmet under his arm; his electric bike was parked outside. In Spanish, he explained he was starting a fever, and that he had a cough and a headache. He thought he had COVID-19, but he was worried about coming to the clinic, as he didn't have insurance. Low-income workers who were most at risk of being exposed to COVID and who were the least protected were also the least likely to have insurance, compounding their vulnerability.

"How much is this visit going to cost me, doc?" he wanted to know.

To my enormous relief, I was able to tell him that *everything* would be covered. He wouldn't have to pay out of pocket for anything.

This was mid-April 2020. By then, Congress had passed the Families First Coronavirus Response Act and the Coronavirus Aid, Relief, and Economic Security Act (CARES), which provided reimbursements on a rolling basis directly to eligible health-care professionals to cover testing and treatment for COVID-19 for uninsured individuals. These were emergency measures designed to account for the fact that people were losing jobs during the pandemic and their health care along with it. People who were uninsured, like this delivery person, and who likely had COVID-19, were now eligible for free testing and treatment. There is no doubt that this emergency measure saved lives. For certain groups of people, it was as if universal health care had finally arrived. Later, we learned that people who lived in states that had already adopted Medicaid expansion under the ACA were much less likely to lose health care in the pandemic. The thirty-one states plus Washington, DC, where health-care coverage was protected during the pandemic thanks to Medicaid expansion included New York, Pennsylvania, and California. The twelve states that have failed to expand Medicaid are all in the South, among them Georgia, Alabama, and Mississippi, and are known to have the worst health outcomes overall as well as the worst racial health inequities.

When the vaccine rollout began, this was also offered to everyone free of charge. At clinics, hospitals, and mobile units across the country, Americans could show up and get their shot without fear of having to pay any out-of-pocket costs. Imagine how US health-care outcomes might change across the board if we could all show up to those same clinics, hospitals, and mobile units and receive free care for whatever ails us, no matter the health con-cern and no matter our insurance status. How many lives might be saved—not to mention how might it reduce health-care costs in a country that spends more money on health care than any other nation on earth, with some of the poorest outcomes com-pared with other high-income nations?

Experts in infectious diseases have long warned that lack of health insurance accelerates the spread of pandemics. If you don't have health insurance, you're likely to delay seeking care, which can place you in danger and can also increase the risk of spread-ing infection to other family members, friends, and colleagues. Most people know that we are the only advanced nation in the world to leave millions of its people without health-care coverage. According to CDC estimates, more than thirty million Ameri-cans were without insurance in the first half of 2021 alone. But not everyone realizes the role that racism has played in prevent-ing us from joining other countries such as Canada and the UK in offering a national health-care service for all.

The closest we came as a nation to a universal health insur-ance provision was after another crisis, World War II. Although private health insurance had been available since the 1920s, this kind of coverage was afforded to only a small number of Ameri-cans and was provided only by employers, but as very few em-ployers offered this benefit—and because Black Americans were usually blocked from applying for or being hired for those jobs that came with such benefits—insurance was for the privileged few. The uninsured had to pay for health care, or simply go with-out. Meanwhile, health-care costs were rising. In the final months of 1945, President Harry S. Truman called on Congress to consider his expanded plan for American health care: a system of national health insurance. His idea was for all Americans to pay fees and taxes each month to cover the cost of a new health-care program that would increase the numbers of trained health-care professionals, expand public health services, increase funding for medical research and education, and lower the cost of medical care.

Truman's plan had broad popular support, with the vast majority of Americans on board. But then the American Medical Association stepped in. At the time, the AMA was the largest and most powerful medical association in the country—and it was also made up of mostly white physicians, due to its ongoing exclusion of and discrimination against Black members from its ranks. When the AMA learned about President Truman's proposals, these white physicians feared that a national health insurance program was going to be bad for profits. They also must have intuited that such a system would mean Black Americans would finally have access to a health-care system that had excluded them since slavery. And so, they launched a strategic campaign to stop Truman's plan in its tracks. The AMA spent millions of dollars on advertisements on the radio and in newspapers and magazines. They sent pamphlets to people's homes. Their message was simple: Keep politics out of medicine. In their literature, they claimed that Truman's plan was "socialized medicine" and "un-American," and that a national health-care system would mean the government officials would now be able to interfere with your health-care decisions. Support for Truman's bill evaporated. Republicans regained control of the House in 1946, marking the bill's death knell. It failed to pass Congress, something that Truman would later cite as the greatest failure of his presidency. Since then, any hope of a national health-care system has been blocked both by the AMA and then by the growing power of private health insurance companies and hospitals. In 2018 alone, health-care companies spent nearly $568 million on lobbying, more than any other industry. Imagine what could be done with that money if it were directed toward actually caring for patients in need.

Black organizations have long been at the forefront of the fight for single-payer, universal health care in this country, because we have always known that having access to health care is a racial justice issue. Despite the AMA's strenuous efforts to crush anything resembling a universal health-care provision, advocacy by organizations such as the National Medical Association, the largest and oldest organization of Black physicians in the US, and Dr. Martin Luther King's Poor People's Campaign continued throughout the 1950s and '60s. The message got out there that health care should be available to everyone, not only those who could afford it. Medicare was established in 1965, a year after the Civil Rights Act was passed, ensuring equitable health care for the elderly. Again, the AMA, a fundamentally racist organization, came out in full force against these changes. But Medicare passed, marking the de facto end of hospital segregation in this country by stipulating that hospitals would not receive federal funding if they continued to segregate.

Medicare and the later passage of Medicaid were landmark moments toward more equitable health care in this country. But they have never been enough. By 2018, the uninsured rate for Black Americans was 11.5 percent, compared with 7.5 percent for whites. For Latinx Americans, the rate was even higher, at 19 percent. Although these rates went down after the Affordable Care Act, inequities remain. Today, Black people are 1.5 times more likely than whites to be without insurance.

This failure to offer free or affordable health care to our citizens has come at a catastrophic cost for decades, particularly during the pandemic. A 2022 study in the journal *Proceedings of the National Academy of Sciences* found, from the pandemic's beginning until mid-March 2022, single-payer, universal health care could have saved more than 338,000 lives from COVID-19 alone. The US could have saved $105.6 billion in health-care costs associated with COVID-19 hospitalizations, in addition to the estimated $438 billion that could be saved in non-pandemic times.

The pandemic has highlighted just how broken our current for-profit health-care system is, leaving far too many people out in the cold to suffer and even die. Would single-payer, universal health care create a more equitable health-care system for everyone? It would be naive to assume it would solve everything. But what we can say, based on systems already in place in this country, is that when health care is provided to every individual, as it is for Medicare patients and veterans through the Veterans Benefits Administration, health outcomes for people of color are substantially improved. If the pandemic taught us anything, it's that we can no longer continue as the only high-income country in the world leaving millions of people without proper access to health care.

As I write this, the protections afforded to vulnerable groups by the pandemic have already been rolled back now that federal funding has run out. Even PCR testing, which was previously free for patients without insurance, is no longer being made available, even to people who are symptomatic. Meanwhile, as we've seen, people who are uninsured are also often likely to be exposed to the virus due to their jobs. In a public health emergency that is far from over, people are still dying preventable deaths every single day. Yet for a little over two years during the pandemic, people like the delivery driver at my clinic got to experience what it felt like to have their COVID-19-related health costs fully covered, even if they couldn't provide an insurance card.

FIFTEEN

THE WAY FORWARD

Actions Speak Louder Than Words

I n March 1955, Dr. Martin Luther King Jr. spoke to a large audience of physicians and health-care workers in Chicago. This was his famous speech in which he decried the American Medical Association and other medical organizations for failing to act to address health-care inequities in the United States. This was the night he spoke the words that form the epigraph to this book: "Of all forms of discrimination and inequalities, injustice in health is the most shocking and inhuman."

For King and so many others like him, health care was a human right that unless enshrined for every citizen would make achieving true equality in the United States an impossibility. In 2023, as I write this, we remain very far from the goal of health care being a human right. Although I wrote this book as a tribute to my mother's legacy and to tell the story of my life and career in medicine, I have ultimately found in the writing that the book is as much about my work and awakening as a physician as it is a call to reimagine who we are as a country. How can we truly be better and do better by those who are most underserved and underestimated by systemic racism? The truth is we need better care infrastructure everywhere—not just in health.

I hope by now you can see the connections among all the systems that work together to oppress Black people. I am calling for Black lives to actually matter. That means Black people deserve access to high-quality, affirming health care, but we also deserve access to economic dignity; access to fair, quality, and affordable housing; access to the best public education and educators of color; the ability to live and thrive free of fear of policing and mass incarceration; a life full of wealth and free of debt given the debts we've already paid; and a chance to gain true generational progress that centers our legacies, our genius, and our contributions.

But to get to this place, our country and our elected and appointed leaders must act courageously and with the will and determination to make our lives better. It's time to stop talking about it and turn empty promises into action. It's time to put our people over punditry—the people who are most affected by racism and injustice often have the best solutions to these ills, because unless you have lived what you *claim* to know and see, you do not deeply understand what so many of us have experienced. It's time we listen and let others lead. That's the way forward.

To My Black Patients and All Black Patients: I'm so sorry the system has failed you. You deserve, at a minimum, dignity and respect. This is not your burden to carry. But I see you if no one else will. You were my motivation for writing this book. I love you.

To Black Physicians and Health-care Professionals: I know exactly how you feel. I've felt isolated. Frustrated. Angry. Sad. I've felt it all. You are not alone. Most of us are doing this work because we care very much about our communities.

Over the past couple of years, I've done deep soul-searching about the role we may play within these institutions and organizations. It's easy because of our socialization, education, and training to become part of the system, but not in a good way. We must be aware that we can even perpetuate harm toward our own patients.

I still don't know where my journey will take me, but I know, for now, I'll work from the outside to make things better on the inside. Remember, you can choose your own path. I truly believe these institutions and organizations do not deserve us, our time, or our labor. We deserve so much better and so do our patients. If you decide to stay, I understand. If you decide to leave, I understand that too.

To Black Women: We are leading so many of the movements to solve our country's most pressing problems, yet we are the most underestimated, disrespected, and disenfranchised group in this country. We cannot keep stepping in to save a nation that doesn't value us. We must find other ways to exist freely, like starting our own ventures on behalf of our communities that will not just rely on change to come from inside the institutions we are working to make better.

Nina Simone said, "You've got to learn to leave the table when love's no longer being served." I believe that deeply.

To Our Black Communities: Our ancestors toiled for a better life in which they would have the freedom to make choices for themselves and their communities. And it is past time for us to bear witness to their dreams. We can replicate what the Black Panthers did in the 1960s, by using a holistic lens to improve health care. Not only did the Panthers open free clinics, but they established free breakfast programs, offered free legal counsel and transportation for families to visit loved ones in prison, and even provided free testing and research for sickle cell disease. We already have organizations in our communities, like the Roots Community Birth Center in north Minneapolis, the Black-owned birthing center I mentioned in chapter nine, which delivers quality and dignified care to Black birthing people by honoring our humanity. We must continue to rely on, support, and love each other.

To People Of Color Who Are Not Black: We need you to recognize that anti-Black racism and white supremacy have pitted us against each other when we should be joining together—and also that anti-Blackness is a global concept. We also need you to understand and appreciate the unique history and experiences of Black people in this country. There is a social hierarchy that places Black people at the very bottom. We need you to have our backs. The civil rights activist and organizer Fannie Lou Hamer said, "Until I am free, you are not free either."

To The Nation's Health-Care Institutions: You have historically, intentionally, and currently proven yourselves untrustworthy to Black communities. You have not treated Black patients with the humanity they deserve. You have excluded community partners in critical decision-making that has affected their neighborhoods and lives. You lack community members on the boards of your institutions. You have not formed meaningful and generative relationships with the community-based organizations that have been embedded in our communities for decades. In your hospital systems, you continue to use race-based tools to calculate, for example, kidney function, and health-care technologies with bias embedded in them, such as pulse oximeters that reinforce and even exacerbate racial health inequities. We need you to do better. We need you to provide structurally competent and culturally centered care to Black communities—care that takes into consideration the social, economic, and political context in which people live. We need you to be intentional about earning the trust of Black communities so that people will be more willing to seek care even before they really need it and have the opportunity to form meaningful and healthy relationships with health-care professionals.

To MEDICAL SCHOOLS AND ACADEMIC MEDICAL CENTERS: You have one of the most important jobs. You are educating our future physicians, but you are not doing enough. I left NYU and many more will leave academic medical centers because of empty and performative diversity statements; creating chief diversity officer or dean of diversity positions that are set up to fail by providing too little commitment in funding, administrative support, and empowerment; your pushback against feedback from Black students, staff, and faculty; and your upholding and relentless centering of white supremacist culture values—like individualism, defensiveness, fear of open conflict, overemphasis of the written word, and quantity over quality—that the educator and activist Dr. Tema Jon Okun has written about so eloquently.

Three things for you to consider:

- First, we need a commitment from you to invest in the pipeline of Black physicians and health-care professionals as early as preschool and engage with children and young people at every step along the path to medical school and beyond. Invest and believe in Black communities—our schools, educational programs, and mentoring—especially considering that many prominent universities directly or indirectly benefited from chattel slavery. Given the profound racial wealth gap in this country, a result of past and current-day systemic racism, you must provide full grants and scholarships for college and medical schools to Black students. You must also specifically engage with those students who are descended from enslaved Black Americans, especially Black American men, whose matriculation rate into medical school has decreased since the 1960s.

- Second, you must commit to a meaningfully diverse, inclusive, and anti-racist learning environment where Black students can show up as their full selves. Listen to students who tell you every day in surveys, interviews, and focus groups what they need to be successful: an environment free of discrimination by their peers and faculty, where they are graded equitably and fairly in their courses and rotations, where the curriculum is taught through a health- and racial-equity lens, where students feel safe to share their lived experiences and to point out what needs to be improved or changed.

- Third, you must not put all the work on the Office of Diversity Affairs or the diversity staff and faculty, or even the students. Our students are attending medical school, and they not only have to focus on their academic obligations but are also forced to lead diversity and anti-racism efforts (which often the schools themselves end up taking credit for), all while confronting racism in society. This feels like violence to us. Every medical school staff, faculty, and leader should have assigned racial equity competencies that they must fulfill in their respective roles, and every role should have anti-racism responsibilities integrated into them. Every individual should feel like the work of dismantling racism is their responsibility.

To White Physicians and Health-care Professionals: This is not our struggle to fight alone. Your Black colleagues are exhausted. Your Black patients are dying. The first step toward fixing racial health inequities is for you to acknowledge that systemic racism exists and do your own due diligence to understand how it operates and impacts health outcomes.

You must recognize your own individual biases and racism, no matter how altruistic or well intentioned you think you are. You may think you are treating all your patients the same, that you are colorblind, that you are giving everyone the best possible care, but you may be reinforcing systemic inequities in your interactions with Black patients by ignoring how interpersonal and systemic racism impact their health.

You must actually do the work of anti-racism beyond reading books and also be held accountable. Self-reflection and training are not enough. Your silence and inaction in the face of racism toward your patients and colleagues is harmful and reflects your complicity. Have you amplified a Black colleague's voice or stepped aside to offer them a leadership role? Did you speak up on behalf of a Black colleague or call out a toxic, racist institutional culture? Are you afraid of rocking the boat and losing your job? The fact is that your Black colleagues and especially your Black patients have so much more to fear than losing a job.

We did not build these institutions, and we do not benefit directly from them.

It's up to you to change them.

To Elected Officials and Leaders: Closing the gap of long-standing racial health inequities will require sustained investment and commitment at all levels of government to dismantle racism and the degree to which it impacts the social determinants of health in Black communities—housing, education, employment, transportation, access to health care and healthy foods, and structural racism within health-care systems.

A checklist, if you will:

- Expand Medicaid in states that have not yet done so to ensure adequate health insurance coverage, and introduce single-payer, universal health coverage to address the high rates of uninsurance and underinsurance in Black communities and provide access to health care.
- Create a revived public health infrastructure and workforce, with funding for workforce training programs for culturally appropriate and responsive workers from Black communities and other communities of color.
- Provide paid sick leave and family and medical leave for all workers—especially those from low-income backgrounds,

and service and essential workers (where Black people are disproportionately represented).

- Ensure the K–12 pipeline for Black physicians and health-care professionals with mentoring opportunities and funding for housing, jobs, and education.

- Allocate funding and resources for adequate housing and opportunities for wealth accumulation in Black communities, given research has shown that eliminating housing segregation would narrow Black-white disparities in income, education, and unemployment. Support access to affordable housing in Black communities—especially in high-opportunity neighborhoods from which Black communities have been traditionally excluded—through expanded federal support for vital affordable-housing and community-development programs.

- Develop equitable housing policies that prioritize Black communities for federal aid and offer direct rental assistance rather than channeling benefits through financial institutions that Black communities are less likely to use.

- To the federal government, we need a long-term and sustained investment for Black communities to reverse the devastation of this pandemic and other pandemics like racism, discrimination, and bias. Since our ancestors were forced onto this soil, for centuries Black communities have been victims of disinvestment and marginalization; the racial health inequities from the COVID-19 pandemic are a direct result of that. We need reparations that give us both the structural and systemic changes we need, as well as wealth-generating strategies and deep ongoing financial commitment to our visions.

To White Americans: You have work to do around your kitchen tables. No more hollow promises. No more ignoring our calls for action. And if you consider yourself liberal or a progressive or a supporter of Black Lives Matter, then that requires you to talk with your family, friends, loved ones, and acquaintances about systemic racism and their own biases, harmful decisions, and silence. Participating in the latest social media hashtag trend does not mean you have reckoned with anything. Our collective grief and the generational and systemic issues we face did not magically appear—white supremacy and privilege have manifested it all.

We are living in two Americas because of systemic racism.

I'm still angry that it took the savage murder of a Black man, George Floyd, by a white police officer for some white Americans to see the horror of racism. He and so many others of us should be alive today, and it should never have taken that heinous incident to wake you up. Anti-Black racism is happening all around you. How will you show up for Black Americans? How will you become a collaborator in dismantling racism? Call out racism and risk losing some relationships. Donate to Black-led racial justice organizations. Interrogate how race, power, and privilege show up in your personal and professional lives. We need you to stop being complacent and comfortable.

If you are a white parent or caregiver, start talking to your children when they're young about race and racism, how it shows up in your and your children's lives, how it harms Black people and other people of color, and then lead by example on how to disrupt racism through your own actions in your personal and professional lives. Your children must learn that racism is not the problem of Black people to solve.

We don't need your guilt; we need your sacrifice and action.

TO THE UNITED STATES: However tragic, depressing, and preventable this current moment is, I also think it's a moment in which we are called upon to think about transformative change more broadly for Black Americans, including how we can and must provide more equitable and quality health care.

If arguably the wealthiest, most well-resourced country in the world cannot take care of its own people, especially those who are crumbling under the weight of oppression, then I am deeply concerned about where we go from here.

I hope that this book is an urgent reminder of the work we have left to do. It takes all of us, from each of our seats on the arc of justice, to make a real difference in people's lives. Beyond rhetoric, we need everyone on board to dismantle systemic racism and white supremacy—these ills are greater than any one of us.

Epilogue

In 1996, my mother contributed to a book of essays about the experiences of women in medical education, written by everyone from female clinicians to basic scientists to administrators. In the book, these physicians shared how being a woman had impacted their personal and professional experiences. In her essay, my mother wrote in detail about growing up in poverty, her decision to pursue a career in medicine, her time at Harvard Medical School and in her residency and fellowship training. Toward the end of the essay, she questioned whether sexism had really been a significant factor in her trajectory.

"In looking back, I believe that many of my negative experiences were as a result of race, not sexism," she wrote. "This is not to minimize the sluggishness of women's progress in medicine, but in this society, race is such a major factor in our actions and policy making that not to acknowledge it is unrealistic and naive."

What my mother wrote in 1996 remains true, appallingly so.

Not only has the percentage of Black physicians failed to increase but numerous racial health inequities have actually worsened since the 1990s. The maternal mortality rate is now higher than it was twenty-five years ago. Black infants are more than twice as likely to die in their first year of life as white infants, a wider inequity now than fifteen years before the end of slavery (although it's important to note that enslavers had a financial interest in keeping Black babies alive because they possessed monetary value). On average, Black men die four years earlier than white men. And from 2019 to 2020, due to the COVID-19 pandemic, Black Americans saw a life expectancy decrease of 2.9 years, while white Americans experienced the smallest decline, of 1.2 years.

I remember the first time I read my mother's essay, at the age of nineteen. It was right after she died, and I had been rummaging through her belongings, trying to find ways to stay connected to her. After I found the book, I read her words greedily, drinking them in, wanting them to comfort me as she used to do so well. But I didn't have the life experience then to truly appreciate what she was writing about. I was unaware of all that she had been through, especially professionally. I was still a college student; I didn't appreciate the complexity of life as time goes on, what happens to you as you get older and have more experiences, taking on more roles. I saw her life story only as one of unremitting triumph, of the little girl who rose up from her humble beginnings to take on the world.

As I sat down to write my own book, I dug out her essay and read it again. I realized, with a jolt, that I was now the same age as she was when she wrote the essay. I was no longer that young woman grieving my mother's recent death. I was a woman in my forties, a physician, and a mother in my own right. Although I still mourned my mother, I was now standing where she had stood. As I read her essay, I realized I no longer saw her story as one of success against the odds. Instead, I was far more aware of the demands that were placed on her as the first person in her family to attend college and then medical school, as a Black physician navigating predominantly white spaces, and as a Black woman juggling motherhood and her career. I could sense her complicated feelings—her passion for medicine, but also her ambivalence because the journey was far from easy. I realized the magnitude of what she had gone through: the lack of food on the table as a child, the absence of a stable home environment, the challenges of coming from a community where few people had walked the same path she was on. The nun who told her she should become a social worker when my mother told her she wanted to be a physician. Being told by a white patient that he did not want to be seen by a Black doctor. I always knew my mother had worked hard and accomplished a lot, but I hadn't always taken into consideration just how exhausting and unnecessary it all was.

"Black people in society learn to develop thick skin," my mother wrote, breaking my heart. "Negative experiences must be turned into positive ones by seeing them as challenges and not insurmountable obstacles. We learn to depend on inner strength to keep us on course. At the present time, for my perseverance, I look to my mother as my role model. I marvel at her just as I marvel at all the black mothers who have achieved the unachievable."

My mother will always be my role model and idol, but it hurts me to know that she had to go through all that she did, to have to overcome all of those barriers. There's the stereotype of the Black superwoman who can do anything and save anyone, even save the world, but it's harmful, especially to Black women. It ignores our humanity—my mother's humanity, my grandmother's humanity. Life shouldn't have been so hard for them. That wasn't fair or just.

Because she died so young, my mother never had a chance to relish all the fruits of her labor, her suffering, her inner strength. I can only imagine how she would have felt the day Oni and I graduated from Harvard Medical School. Although our mother wasn't there that day, our self-appointed godmother, who had been best friends with our maternal grandmother—a warm, exuberant elderly woman named Miss Alleyne—was in the crowd to support us alongside the rest of our family members. Miss Alleyne, an ordained minister, was born in rural Alabama, and she had cared for my mother when she was sick, driving her to and from her chemotherapy appointments and preparing her meals. As Oni's name was called, immediately followed by mine, and we walked proudly across the stage, I could hear someone wailing my mother's name:

"Daaaaale! Daaaaale! Yo' babies! Yo' babies!!!"

I looked out into the audience, squinted, and in the distance saw my family on either side of Miss Alleyne, attempting to hold her up as she wept uncontrollably.

"Daaaaale! Daaaaale!" she called out.

Miss Alleyne deeply understood the magnitude of what was happening in that moment, the generations of struggle and perseverance that got Oni and me to that stage that day.

When Oni and I graduated Harvard Medical School, there were

various tributes paid to us as the "first Black mother-daughter legacy." The message was that we had triumphed, and we should be celebrated for that. But for us, the word *legacy* means something different. Yes, it's a celebration of our mother's hard work—in her career as a physician and in her personal life as a parent—but it's also an acknowledgment that systemic racism makes the whole journey harder for us. Accessing resources and opportunities to apply to medical school is harder, staying the course is harder, finding mentorship and sponsorship is harder; so it's not the same as white legacy by any means. For us, *legacy* is a tribute to our mother, an acknowledgment of the barriers she was forced to overcome and a lifelong commitment to making the way easier for those in the future.

I can only imagine how my mother's life might have unfolded had she been given more time. Before she got sick, she had plans. Faced with her empty nest, she was making changes. She was considering going back to school for a master's degree in public health; becoming triple boarded in internal medicine, nephrology, and geriatrics still wasn't enough for her. And she had waited until we were off at college to make the difficult decision to ask my father for a divorce after their decades-long marriage. She was at a moment in her personal and professional life when she was deciding what would be next for her, right on the brink of reclaiming her life on her own terms, before she had to stop everything to focus on the treatment.

"Am I satisfied I went into medicine?" my mother asks in the essay. "Were there different pressures on me as a minority woman in medicine? Would I do things differently if I had to do things over today?" Those are the same questions I asked myself before I left NYU. Did I even want to stay in academic medicine? Would I be able to reach my fullest potential in a conservative, predominantly white environment? Did I need to think differently about my life and career and about what success looks like? As a younger woman I didn't internalize what she was saying, but reading her essay thirty years later, her words could almost be mine.

These days, I even wonder if I would want my children to pursue careers in medicine. As I write this, they are six and eight years old, still young and innocent. When I think about the stress and trauma of racism they would experience as Black men entering the medical realm, my answer would be no. I want to protect them. I worry that a career in medicine would be like throwing them to the wolves. I don't have the same drive for traditional notions of success that our mother had for Oni and me. As someone who was born into poverty, our mother wanted and needed something very different for her daughters. My children have had the kind of privileged life every Black child deserves, but I would prefer for them to consider all the possibilities for how they might live full and fulfilling lives. My children deserve that.

Even though my children are still young, my life has surpassed my mother's in some ways. I have gone down the road she didn't get to go down. I have ended my marriage; I have found my voice outside of medicine as a health equity advocate and social impact entrepreneur. Even though she didn't get to have those experiences, I still consider myself lucky to have the example of someone who wanted to do that for herself. I've gotten to do it for her—and for myself. I learned from her early death that life is unpredictable, and you have to take chances. In fact, you must take chances.

The same determination that motivated her drives me to continue where she left off, to use my voice in ways that I never thought I would or could, and to take a leap of faith because I knew in my heart I could make a larger impact on the issues that are important to me, to us, to our communities. Despite the challenges of her own journey, my mother finished her essay with words of affirmation: "I am honored to be a physician. That little six-year-old girl sitting in the welfare center would never have dreamed that one day she would become a physician, let alone know what a physician was."

Our mother had grown up without access to health care, not understanding what a physician was. Thanks to her, Oni and I never had to imagine what health care looked like, or what the job of a physician entailed. As little girls, we got to play with her doctor's bag, visit her at the hospital, and watch her as she cared for her patients. Our mother exposed us to the possibility that we could be physicians too, and that was incredibly powerful, to see someone you love and admire doing this work. She cleared a path for us, so that all we had to do was follow in her wake.

After she died, Oni and I inherited her old black doctor's bag with her name written in gold on the side. We're still running with it.

ACKNOWLEDGMENTS

During August 2020, I received an email that started me on the journey of writing *Legacy*.

It was from Neeti Madan, a book agent with Sterling Lord Literistic. She wrote, "I've been reading your essays, Twitter posts, and most recently heard you on NPR. I wonder if you have considered writing and publishing a book, as I—along with many others, I am sure—am always impressed and intrigued by your professional and personal perspectives on important issues."

I found out later that Neeti had been on vacation at her mother's house and had heard me speaking as a guest on one of my favorite shows, WNYC's *The Brian Lehrer Show*. After my segment, she sent me a lovely email and the rest is history. That story reminds me that even when you think people are not listening to you, they really are, and you never know who is listening. You must keep speaking up.

Writing *Legacy* has been a once-in-a-lifetime opportunity, a labor of love, and a journey through self-discovery all bundled in one. I had to directly confront the grief from my beloved mother's premature death, and my decision to leave academic medicine—one that I never thought I would ever have to make, and my anger at the horrific way that Black people have been physically and psychologically harmed by living in this country. I laid myself bare. I told deeply personal stories about my family, my patients, and my career.

I could not have gotten to this point in my life without my inspirations and my village. Some are the people who I have connected and formed relationships with since I was a child and at various stages in my life. Many have either loved, supported, sponsored, or mentored me. Others are scholars or intellectuals whose work I have deeply admired and have inspired my own life and career.

To my nursery school, Little Sun People, and its founder and director, Fela Barclift, aka Mama Fela, I feel incredibly lucky that LSP provided the strong foundation and love that Oni and I needed as little Black children growing up in Brooklyn. Our experience at LSP was and continues to be integral to our identity as a Black Americans.

To my teachers and the administration at my elementary school, St. Mark's Day School, thank you for investing in us children from Brooklyn's Black and Afro-Caribbean families. I learned the words to "Lift Every Voice and Sing" before I was in the first grade, and sang it proudly with my head held high every single time. To Vonetta, Adeola, Taiwo, Aisha, Hakim, Hanif, Shani, and so many more, I'm grateful to have had the honor of growing up in 1980s Brooklyn with you.

To my classmates in the Stuyvesant Class of 1995, the Harvard College Class of 1999, and the Harvard Medical School Class of 2005, thank you for your friendship and support.

To the Black women physicians who I was surrounded by as a child, including Dr. Mildred Clarke, Dr. June Mulvaney, and the other members of the Susan Smith McKinney Steward Medical Society and the Provident Clinical Society, you were and remain the blueprint for me. To mother's HMS classmates Dr. Jessie Sherrod, Dr. Mary Flowers, and others, you continue to be an inspiration to me. As a child, I thought Black women physicians made up most physicians. I didn't realize until I was in my teens that wasn't the case. Because of you, I always knew I could be Dr. Blackstock.

To Harvard Medical School's Office of Recruitment and Multicultural Affairs, especially Dr. Alvin Poussaint, Rosa Soler, and Beverlee Turner, you have my deepest gratitude for creating a space at HMS where we could always feel safe, supported, and loved. To Dr. Ronald Arky, thank you for your kindness and interest in my overall well-being during medical school.

To my senior residents and my attendings at Kings County Hospital and SUNY Downstate Department of Emergency Medicine, especially Rob Gore, Reinaldo Austin, Claritza Rios, Dara Kass, Elma Johnson, Jonathan Wasserman, Stephan Rinnert, Chris Doty, Shahriar Zehtabchi, Sigrid Wolfram, and Jessica Stetz, thank you for your guidance and mentoring. Thank you for believing in me.

To my former NYU students and residents, especially Natasha, Kamini, Adaira, Tsion, Tunmise, and Gladyne, I love you all so much and can't wait to see what wonderful ways you improve this world.

To The OpEd Project and Katie Orenstein, thank you for helping me find my voice. Taking your one-day workshop on writing op-eds changed my life.

To Lachelle Dawn, thank you for taking the time to speak with me about blood cancers, and specifically myelodysplastic syndrome and acute myelogenous leukemia. Your perspective has enriched this book.

To Rachel Hardeman, sis, thank you for everything—your scholarship, your expertise, and your kindness. The work that you do is so incredibly invaluable. Everyone should know it.

To Sirry Alang, one of the loveliest human beings who I've never met, thank you for your kindness, your scholarship, and just being you. You inspire me in ways that I could never fully explain, but at the most basic, you make me brave. I love the love that you and Uju create and only wish the very best for both of you.

To the following scholars, journalists, and notable individuals, bell hooks, Shirley Chisolm, Audre Lorde, Tema Okun, Harriet A. Washington, Lisa Cooper, Deidra Crews, David R. Williams, Dorothy Roberts, Camara Jones, Jonathan Metzl, and Helena Hansen, your words and work have inspired my personal life and career.

To Black women-led organizations and leaders, like Chanel Porchia-

Albert of Ancient Song Doula Services; Joia Crear-Perry, founder of National Birth Equity Collective; Kiddada Green, founding executive director of Black Mothers' Breastfeeding Association; and Rebecca Polson, owner and director of the Roots Community Birth Center, thank you for leading the way.

To Takirra, Maia, and Monnikue of Unapologetic Communications, thank you for supporting me and all the work that I've done since we have connected. Thank you for teaching me to be an unapologetic Black woman.

To Traci, my talent agent, I still can't believe you found me during one of my first MSNBC appearances when I didn't know how to apply makeup and I was wearing a frumpy dress, but you immediately saw my passion and knew what I was about. Thank you as always for your support, advocacy, and friendship.

To my Twitter fam, including Taison, Utibe, Max, Anna, Alfiee, Lena G., Alycia W., Rebecca C., Zoe M., Kim C., Nick S.F., Stella, Ijeoma N.O, Ijeoma O., Vanessa G., Danté, Raven, Brian L., David M., Kaliris, Tiffany, Saskia, Robin, and so many more, thank you for always showing me love and having my back.

To my chosen family over the years, Dana, Nicole, Dzifa, Helen, Ediri, Kalyani, Marie, Renee, Danice, Julene, Ola, Tolu, Jane, Ofole, Joella, Crystal, Rhonda, Brandi, Addy, Valesia, Lesley, Elsa, Aisha and Stephanie, I love you.

To the Viking team—Andrea Schulz, vice president and editor in chief; Associate Publisher Kate Stark; Lindsay Prevette, director of publicity; and Assistant Editor Camille LeBlanc, thank you for believing in *Legacy* and seeing the vision for what a powerful and transformative book that it could ultimately become.

To Allison Lorentzen, my executive editor, I knew from the first time we met that you got me. I knew that you saw me. I knew that I would be able to tell this story in the most authentic way if we worked together. I still reread the letter you sent me after our first intro call. I feel lucky that we are now connected.

To Neeti, my book agent, ever since we first spoke by phone, I knew that I wanted you to be my agent. Working with you is not only fun but I also value your sage perspective and your friendship. I love being on this journey with you and I hope we'll have many more opportunities to work together.

To Eve, I'll miss our weekly meetings. Your perspective during the writing process was invaluable and made *Legacy* so very rich.

To Rolisa, thank you for keeping me sane and being my protector. I cherish our personal and professional relationship very much and I look forward to working together for many more years to come.

To my Advancing Health Equity team, what would I do without you all? Samantha, Candice, ChiChi, Jess, Tiffany, Kellie, Angelique, and Shannon, I'm beyond grateful for you all and it's an honor to work with you.

To my extended family, Ms. Alleyne, Mama Del, Brother Orlendo, Auntie Paula, and Pamela, thank you for taking care of my parents, Oni, and me during the most challenging times. I love you all very much.

To Valentine, Nicole, Lisette, and Tracy, thank you for loving and caring for the boys so that I can be the best mama to them.

To CJR and the Rose family, I know you think nothing of it, but that I know the boys are being taken care of and doted on in the most loving way when they aren't with me is one of the reasons I could find the peace to write this book. CJR, the boys are lucky to have you as their father.

To my Auntie Joanie and Uncle Michael, I know we are no longer in touch, but you two were such huge parts of my happy childhood. I hope that one day we can connect again. I only hope and want good things for both of you.

To Shanequa, I'm beyond grateful that I found you and that Oni connected us. Having the opportunity to sit down and talk with you twice a month is a gift that I will always be profoundly grateful for. Thank you for keeping me sane and grounded over the last five years.

To my father, Daddy, I remember visiting Clarendon, Jamaica, as a little girl with you and being shocked to see where you grew up. Thank you for making sure we lived in our own beautiful home, that we went to schools where we would thrive, and for always waiting for us late at night as kids to pick us up from parties so that we were safe. I hope we have a chance in this lifetime or maybe the next to understand each other a little more. I do love you very much, Daddy, and I'm glad that you and Shirley can spend some good times together in your remaining years. To Michelle and Marcia, sending love to both of you.

To my mother, Mommy, I love you deeply. I miss you terribly. I miss your hugs and kisses. I miss your voice. I miss our long conversations. I miss your smile. I thought that the pain of your death would go away, but instead it's turned into numbness. There were so many experiences we were supposed to have together. I will never get over your premature death and the suffering you endured, but I know that *Legacy* will make you proud.

To my original wombmate, my twin sister, Oni. I love you to the moon and back. You are one of the most brilliant and thoughtful people I know. I don't take your love for granted. I could not have written *Legacy* without your eyes, your time, and your perspective. *Legacy* could not have been the gift it is without you. I'm immensely grateful to you, Sweets.

Finally, my two children, becoming your mama has been one of the most humbling, hardest, and most beautiful experiences of my life. I want this world to be better because of you. I worry about having to leave you eventually, but my goal is to make sure you have skills to thrive and to lead a content life. Thank you for your sweet love, kisses, and hugs. I'm absolutely smitten with you.

Thank you to everyone who has taken the time to read *Legacy* and open your hearts and minds to making this country a more equitable and just place.

NOTES

INTRODUCTION

4 **One of the promises:** Monika K. Goyal et al., "Racial Disparities in Pain Management of Children with Appendicitis in Emergency Departments," *JAMA Pediatrics* 169, no. 11 (2015): 996–1002, doi.org/10.1001/jamapediatrics.2015.1915; Carmen R. Green et al., "The Unequal Burden of Pain: Confronting Racial and Ethnic Disparities in Pain," *Pain Medicine* 4, no. 3 (2003): 277–94, doi.org/10.1046/j.1526-4637.2003.03034.x; Knox H. Todd et al., "Ethnicity and Analgesic Practice," *Annals of Emergency Medicine* 35, no. 1 (2000): 11–6, doi.org/10.1016/S0196-0644(00)70099-0.

5 **Studies indicate that Black babies:** Brad N. Greenwood et al., "Physician-Patient Racial Concordance and Disparities in Birthing Mortality for Newborns," *Proceedings of the National Academy of Sciences* 117, no. 35 (2020): 21194–200, doi.org/10.1073/pnas.1913405117.

5 **What's more, Black physicians:** Miriam Komaromy et al., "The Role of Black and Hispanic Physicians in Providing Health Care for Underserved Populations," *New England Journal of Medicine* 334 (1996): 1305–10, https://doi.org/10.1056/NEJM199605163342006; Lyndonna M. Marrast et al., "Minority Physicians' Role in the Care of Underserved Patients: Diversifying the Physician Workforce May Be Key in Addressing Health Disparities," *JAMA Internal Medicine* 174, no. 2 (2014): 289–91, doi.org/10.1001/jamainternmed.2013.12756; Imam M. Xierali and Marc A. Nivet, "The Racial and Ethnic Composition and Distribution of Primary Care Physicians," *Journal of Health Care for the Poor and Underserved* 29, no. 1 (2018): 556–70, doi.org/10.1353/hpu.2018.0036.

279

5 **The number of Black:** Dan P. Ly, "Historical Trends in the Representativeness and Incomes of Black Physicians, 1900–2018," *Journal of General Internal Medicine* 37 (2021): 1310–2, doi.org/10.1007/s11606-021-06745-1.

6 **US data collection:** D. L. Hoyert, "Maternal Mortality and Related Concepts," *Vital and Health Statistics* 3, no. 33, National Center for Health Statistics (2007), cdc.gov/nchs/data/series/sr_03/sr03_033.pdf.

6 **At that time, Black:** Eugene Declercq and Laurie Zephyrin, "Maternal Mortality in the United States: A Primer," Commonwealth Fund, December 16, 2020, doi.org/10.26099/talq-mw24.

6 **Currently, Black men:** Elizabeth Arias, Betzaida Tejada-Vera, and Farida Ahmad, "Provisional Life Expectancy Estimates for January through June, 2020," *National Center for Health Statistics* 10 (2021), dx.doi.org/10.15620/cdc:100392.

6 **Black babies have:** Danielle M. Ely and Anne K. Driscoll, "Infant Mortality in the United States, 2018: Data from the Period Linked Birth/Infant Death File," *National Center for Health Statistics* 69, no. 7 (2020), cdc.gov/nchs/data/nvsr/nvsr69/NVSR-69-7-508.pdf.

7 **Even with my:** "Racial/Ethnic Disparities in Pregnancy-Related Deaths—United States, 2007–2016," Centers for Disease Control and Prevention, accessed December 5, 2022, cdc.gov/reproductivehealth/maternal-mortality/disparities-pregnancy-related-deaths/Infographic-disparities-pregnancy-related-deaths-h.pdf.

8 **The framework of structural competency:** Jonathan M. Metzl and Helena Hansen, "Structural Competency: Theorizing a New Medical Engagement with Stigma and Inequality," *Social Science & Medicine* 103 (2014): 126–33, doi.org/10.1016/j.socscimed.2013.06.032.

CHAPTER 1   THE ORIGINAL DR. BLACKSTOCK

17 **But I believe she:** "Race, Ethnicity, & Kidney Disease," National Institute of Diabetes and Digestive and Kidney Diseases, accessed December 5, 2022, niddk.nih.gov/health-information/kidney-disease/race-ethnicity.

24 **For centuries in this country:** Ann Steinecke and Charles Terrell, "Progress for Whose Future? The Impact of the Flexner Report on Medical Education for Racial and Ethnic Minority Physicians in the United States," *Academic Medicine* 85, no. 2 (2010): 236–45, doi.org/10.1097/ACM.0b013e3181c885be.

24 **It was only after the:** "African American Physicians and Organized Medicine, 1846–1968," American Medical Association, accessed December 5, 2022, ama-assn.org/sites/ama-assn.org/files/corp/media-browser/public/ama-history/african-american-physicians-organized-medicine-timeline.pdf.

26 **And it wasn't until:** "Black History Month: A Medical Perspective: Education," Duke University Medical Center Library and Archives, last updated October 20, 2022, guides.mclibrary.duke.edu/blackhistorymonth/education.

26 **The reason was the publication:** Elizabeth Hlavinka, "Racial Bias in

Flexner Report Permeates Medical Education Today," *MedPage Today,* June 18, 2020, medpagetoday.com/publichealthpolicy/medicaleducation /87171.

27 **"Not only does":** Terri Laws, "How Should We Respond to Racist Legacies in Health Professions Education Originating in the Flexner Report?" *American Medical Association Journal of Ethics* 23, no. 3 (2021): 271–5, https://doi.org/10.1001/amajethics.2021.271; Abraham Flexner, "Medical Education in the United States and Canada," *Science* 32, no. 810 (1910): 41–50, doi.org/10.1126/science.32.810.41.

27 **Almost a hundred:** Kendall M. Campbell et al., "Projected Estimates of African American Medical Graduates of Closed Historically Black Medical Schools," *JAMA Network Open* 3, no. 8 (2020): e2015220, doi.org/10.1001 /jamanetworkopen.2020.15220.

28 **For context, in 2015:** Hector Mora et al., "The National Deficit of Black and Hispanic Physicians in the US and Projected Estimates of Time to Correction," *JAMA Network Open* 5, no. 6 (2022): e2215485, doi:10.1001 /jamanetworkopen.2022.15485.

29 **The modern MCAT:** Catherine Reinis Lucey and Aaron Saguil, "The Consequences of Structural Racism on MCAT Scores and Medical School Admissions: The Past Is Prologue," *Academic Medicine* 95, no. 3 (2020): 351–6, doi.org/10.1097/ACM.0000000000002939.

29 **Studies have shown that election:** Dowin Boatright et al., "Racial Disparities in Medical Student Membership in the Alpha Omega Alpha Honor Society," *JAMA Internal Medicine* 177, no. 5 (2017): 659–65, doi.org/10 .1001/jamainternmed.2016.9623.

29 **Because academic medical:** Mark C. Henderson, Charlene Green, and Candice Chen, "What Does It Mean for Medical School Admissions to Be Socially Accountable?" *American Medical Association Journal of Ethics* 23, no. 12 (2021): 965–74, doi.org/10.1001/amajethics.2021.965.

CHAPTER 2 SOMETHING WRONG

42 **The same year my:** Office of the Comptroller of the Currency, "Community Developments Fact Sheet: Community Reinvestment Act," 2014, occ.gov /publications-and-resources/publications/community-affairs/community -developments-fact-sheets/pub-fact-sheet-cra-reinvestment-act-mar -2014.pdf.

44 **What I didn't know:** Lindsey Rae Gjording, "Redlining and Its Impact on New York City," *CitySignal,* October 25, 2022, citysignal.com/redlining -and-its-impact-on-new-york-city/.

45 **In 1944, the GI:** Erin Blakemore, "How the GI Bill's Promise Was Denied to a Million Black WWII Veterans," History, April 20, 2021, history.com /news/gi-bill-black-wwii-veterans-benefits.

46 **The legacy and impact:** Julia Perrino, "'Redlining' and Health Indicators:

Decisions Made 80 Years Ago Have Health Consequences Today," National Community Reinvestment Coalition, July 2, 2020, ncrc.org/redlining-and -health-indicators-decisions-made-80-years-ago-have-health -consequences-today/.

46 **This meant the people living:** Maria Godoy, "In U.S. Cities, the Health Effects of Past Housing Discrimination Are Plain to See," NPR, November 19, 2020, npr.org/sections/health-shots/2020/11/19/911909187/in-u-s-cities -the-health-effects-of-past-housing-discrimination-are-plain-to-see.

46 **Another study, conducted:** Meg Anderson, "Racist Housing Practices from the 1930s Linked to Hotter Neighborhoods Today," NPR, January 14, 2020, npr.org/2020/01/14/795961381/racist-housing-practices-from-the -1930s-linked-to-hotter-neighborhoods-today.

48 **Studies show that people like my father:** Tod G. Hamilton and Tiffany L. Green, "From the West Indies to Africa: A Universal Generational Decline in Health among Blacks in the United States," *Social Science Research* 73 (2018): 163–74, doi.org/10.1016/j.ssresearch.2017.12.003.

CHAPTER 3   EVERYTHING WE LOST

55 **Today, there are four:** Ari Ephraim Feldman, "New York City Now Has Four Superfund Sites. Where Are They?" *Spectrum News NY1*, April 22, 2022, ny1.com/nyc/all-boroughs/news/2022/04/21/new-york-city-now-has -four-superfund-sites--where-are-they-.

55 **Multiple studies show that people:** Vann R. Newkirk II, "Trump's EPA Concludes Environmental Racism Is Real," *Atlantic*, February 28, 2018, theatlantic.com/politics/archive/2018/02/the-trump-administration-finds -that-environmental-racism-is-real/554315/.

55 **We also know that these high rates:** "Cancer Disparities in the Black Community," American Cancer Society, accessed December 5, 2022, cancer .org/about-us/what-we-do/health-equity/cancer-disparities-in-the-black -community.html; Robert W. Carlson, "Treatment Barriers Create Racial Disparities in Cancer Care. They Need to Come Down," *STAT*, June 24, 2020, statnews.com/2020/06/24/cancer-care-racial-disparities-dismantle -barriers/; Ola Landgren, "Racial/Ethnic Disparities: Need More Work!" *Blood* 130, no. 15 (2017): 1685–6, doi.org/10.1182/blood-2017-08-798546.

56 **Recent studies point:** Christopher M. Aldrighetti et al., "Racial and Ethnic Disparities among Participants in Precision Oncology Clinical Studies," *JAMA Network Open* 4, no. 11 (2021): e2133205, doi.org/10.1001 /jamanetworkopen.2021.33205.

56 **Aging is another key:** "Risk Factors for Acute Myeloid Leukemia (AML)," American Cancer Society, accessed December 5, 2022, cancer.org/cancer /acute-myeloid-leukemia/causes-risks-prevention/risk-factors.html.

57 **Studies have shown that the higher:** Gene Demby, "Making the Case That Discrimination Is Bad for Your Health," *Code Switch Podcast*, NPR, Janu-

ary 14, 2018, npr.org/sections/codeswitch/2018/01/14/577664626/making
-the-case-that-discrimination-is-bad-for-your-health.

57 **This phenomenon has:** Arline T. Geronimus and Sanders Korenman,
"Maternal Youth or Family Background? On the Health Disadvantages of
Infants with Teenage Mothers," *American Journal of Epidemiology* 137, no.
2 (1993): 213–25, doi.org/10.1093/oxfordjournals.aje.a116662.

58 **Today, the National Cancer:** Kedar Kirtane and Stephanie J. Lee, "Racial
and Ethnic Disparities in Hematologic Malignancies," *Blood* 130, no. 15
(2017): 1699–705, doi.org/10.1182/blood-2017-04-778225.

CHAPTER 4 ALL THE THINGS THEY DIDN'T TEACH ME

71 **No one ever spoke:** Ayah Nuriddin, Graham Mooney, and Alexandre I. R.
White, "Reckoning with Histories of Medical Racism and Violence in the
USA," *Lancet* 396, no. 10256 (2020): 949–51, doi.org/10.1016/S0140-6736
(20)32032-8.

71 **Both Northern and Southern:** Daina Ramey Berry, "Beyond the Slave
Trade, the Cadaver Trade," *New York Times*, February 3, 2018, nytimes.com
/2018/02/03/opinion/sunday/cadavers-slavery-medical-schools.html.

72 **As Skloot describes:** Leah Samuel, "5 important Ways Henrietta Lacks
Changed Medical Science," *STAT*, April 14, 2017, statnews.com/2017/04
/14/henrietta-lacks-hela-cells-science/.

72 **Of note, Skloot:** Steve Hendrix, "On the Eve of an Oprah Movie about Henrietta Lacks, an Ugly Feud Consumes the Familly," *Washington Post*, March
29, 2017, washingtonpost.com/local/on-the-eve-of-an-oprah-movie-about
-henrietta-lacks-an-ugly-feud-consumes-the-family/2017/03/28/d33d3418
-1248-11e7-ada0-1489b735b3a3_story.html.

73 **But no one ever taught us:** Sarah Zhang, "The Surgeon Who Experimented
on Slaves," *Atlantic*, April 18, 2018, theatlantic.com/health/archive/2018
/04/j-marion-sims/558248/.

73 **At medical school we were taught:** Ike Swetlitz, "Mistrust after Tuskegee
Experiments May Have Taken Years off Black Men's Lives," *STAT*, June 16,
2016, statnews.com/2016/06/16/mistrust-tuskegee-black-men/.

75 **Much later in:** Usha Lee McFarling, "Expert Panel Recommends against
Use of Race in Assessment of Kidney Function," *STAT*, September 23, 2021,
statnews.com/2021/09/23/expert-panel-recommends-against-use-of-race
-based-tool-in-assessment-of-kidney-function/.

76 **Enslavers found willing:** Paul Erickson, "The Anthropology of Charles
Caldwell, M.D." *Isis* 72, no. 2 (1981): 252–6, http://www.jstor.org/stable
/230972; Karina Chowdhury and Erin Fanning Madden, "Scientific Racism
Attitudes among Diverse Undergraduate Pre–Health Professions Students,"
Pedagogy in Health Promotion 7, no. 4 (2021): 331–40, doi.org/10.1177
/23733799211043136.

77 **In fact, the pulmonary:** Linda Villarosa, "Myths about Physical Racial

Differences Were Used to Justify Slavery—and Are Still Believed by Doctors Today," *New York Times Magazine*, August 14, 2019, nytimes.com/interactive /2019/08/14/magazine/racial-differences-doctors.html.

77 **In the 1820s, Dr. Thomas Hamilton:** Villarosa, "Myths about Physical Racial Differences Were Used to Justify Slavery."

78 **Instead, according to:** Ike Swetlitz, "Some Medical Students Still Think Black Patients Feel Less Pain Than Whites," *STAT*, April 4, 2016, statnews .com/2016/04/04/medical-students-beliefs-race-pain/; Kelly M. Hoffman et al., "Racial Bias in Pain Assessment and Treatment Recommendations, and False Beliefs about Biological Differences between Blacks and Whites," *Proceedings of the National Academy of Sciences* 113, no. 16 (2016): 4296–301, doi.org/10.1073/pnas.1516047113.

CHAPTER 5   MISDIAGNOSED

88 **Certainly, it's not:** Prashant Mahajan et al., "Factors Associated with Potentially Missed Diagnosis of Appendicitis in the Emergency Department," *JAMA Network Open* 3, no. 3 (2020): e200612, doi.org/10.1001 /jamanetworkopen.2020.0612.

88 **Negative images or:** Lisa Rosenthal and Marci Lobel, "Stereotypes of Black American Women Related to Sexuality and Motherhood," *Psychology of Women Quarterly* 40, no. 3 (2016): 414–27, doi.org/10.1177 /0361684315627459.

90 **A 2016 report:** Julie Onos, "Race and Medicine: The Cost of Medical Bias When You're Sick, Black, and Female," Healthline, September 30, 2020, healthline.com/health/the-cost-of-medical-bias-when-youre-sick-black -and-female#1.

90 **The meta-analysis of:** Janice A. Sabin, "How We Fail Black Patients in Pain," Association of American Medical Colleges, January 6, 2020, aamc.org /news-insights/how-we-fail-black-patients-pain.

90 **A 2020 study:** Monika K. Goyal et al., "Racial and Ethnic Differences in Emergency Department Pain Management of Children with Fractures," *Pediatrics* 145, no. 5 (2020): doi.org/10.1542/peds.2019-3370.

CHAPTER 6   HOMECOMING

96 **Because the US:** Samantha Artiga et al., "Health Coverage by Race and Ethnicity, 2010–2021," KFF, December 20, 2022, kff.org/racial-equity -and-health-policy/issue-brief/health-coverage-by-race-and-ethnicity/.

97 **Prior to the 1960s:** Vann R. Newkirk II, "America's Health Segregation Problem," *Atlantic*, May 18, 2016, theatlantic.com/politics/archive/2016 /05/americas-health-segregation-problem/483219/.

97 **The first ever:** Brian J. Zink, "Social Justice, Egalitarianism, and the History of Emergency Medicine," *American Medical Association Journal of*

Ethics 12, no. 6 (2010): 492–4, doi.org/10.1001/virtualmentor.2010.12
.6.mhstl-1006.

98 **That changed in 1967:** Bill O'Driscoll, "How Working-Class Black Men in Pittsburgh Pioneered Emergency Medicine," *Morning Edition*, NPR, September 20, 2022, npr.org/2022/09/20/1124008613/how-working-class -black-men-in-pittsburgh-pioneered-emergency-medicine; Matthew L. Edwards, "Race, Policing, and History—Remembering the Freedom House Ambulance Service," *New England Journal of Medicine* 384 (2021): 1386–9, doi.org/10.1056/NEJMp2035467.

99 **Today, nearly half:** University of Maryland School of Medicine, "Nearly Half of US Medical Care Comes from Emergency Rooms," *ScienceDaily*, October 17, 2017, sciencedaily.com/releases/2017/10/171017091849.htm.

104 **A 2017 study:** University of Maryland School of Medicine, "Nearly Half of US Medical Care Comes from Emergency Rooms."

105 **In 2006, when:** Joseph Mantone, "Operating Deficit Grows at N.Y.C. Public System," *Modern Healthcare*, March 13, 2006, modernhealthcare.com /article/20060313/NEWS/603130332/operating-deficit-grows-at-n-y-c -public-system; Sewell Chan, "City Hospitals May Need More Aid to Counter Deficit," *New York Times*, March 13, 2006, nytimes.com/2006/03 /13/nyregion/city-hospitals-may-need-more-aid-to-counter-deficit.html.

CHAPTER 7   THREE PATIENTS

114 **Sickle cell is an incurable:** S. G. Damle, "New Hope in Fight against Sickle Cell Anemia?" *Contemporary Clinical Dentistry* 8, no. 1 (2017): 1–2, doi.org /10.4103/ccd.ccd_275_17.

114 **Today, there are one hundred thousand:** "Data & Statistics on Sickle Cell Disease," Centers for Disease Control and Prevention, last modified May 2, 2022, cdc.gov/ncbddd/sicklecell/data.html.

117 **In one recent study:** Sharon Begley, "'Every Time It's a Battle': In Excruciating Pain, Sickle Cell Patients Are Shunted Aside," *STAT*, September 18, 2017, statnews.com/2017/09/18/sickle-cell-pain-treatment/.

117 **In another study, led:** Paula Tanabe et al., "Evaluation of a Train-the-Trainer Workshop on Sickle Cell Disease for ED Providers," *Journal of Emergency Nursing* 39, no. 6 (2013): 539–46, doi.org/10.1016/j.jen.2011.05.010.

117 **In another study, researchers:** Carlton Haywood Jr. et al., "The Impact of Race and Disease on Sickle Cell Patient Wait Times in the Emergency Department," *American Journal of Emergency Medicine* 31, no. 4 (2013): 651–6, doi.org/10.1016/j.ajem.2012.11.005.

118 **Sickle cell anemia was first:** Paul S. Frenette and George F. Atweh, "Sickle Cell Disease: Old Discoveries, New Concepts, and Future Promise," *Journal of Clinical Investigation* 117, no. 4 (2007): 850–8, doi.org/10.1172 /JCI30920.

118 **Because it's perceived as:** Sharon Begley, "We've Known for 50 Years

What Causes Sickle Cell Disease. Where's the Cure?" *STAT,* May 19, 2016, https://www.statnews.com/2016/05/19/sickle-cell-disease-cure/; Sharon Begley, "With a Rapper's Death, Harsh Spotlight Falls on Slow Progress against Sickle Cell," *STAT,* June 21, 2017, statnews.com/2017/06/21/prodigy -sickle-cell/.

118 **There are 28 drugs:** Jenny Gold, "Miracle of Hemophilia Drugs Comes at a Steep Price," NPR, March 5, 2018, npr.org/sections/health-shots/2018/03 /05/589469361/miracle-of-hemophilia-drugs-comes-at-a-steep-price.

118 **Cystic fibrosis affects:** Faheem Farooq et al., "Comparison of US Federal and Foundation Funding of Research for Sickle Cell Disease and Cystic Fibrosis and Factors Associated with Research Productivity," *JAMA Network Open* 3, no. 3 (2020): e201737, doi.org/10.1001/jamanetworkopen.2020.1737.

118 **In the early 1970s:** Mary T. Bassett, "Beyond Berets: The Black Panthers as Health Activists," *American Journal of Public Health* 106, no. 10 (2016): 1741–3, doi.org/10.2105/AJPH.2016.303412; Alondra Nelson, *Body and Soul: The Black Panther Party and the Fight against Medical Discrimination* (Minneapolis: University of Minnesota Press, 2011), 115–52.

122 **Studies show that Black women:** Elizabeth Czukas, "Why Do Black Women Experience More Pregnancy Loss?" Verywell Family, April 24, 2021, verywell-family.com/why-do-black-women-have-more-pregnancy-losses-2371724.

122 **A 2013 study:** Sudeshna Mukherjee et al., "Risk of Miscarriage among Black Women and White Women in a US Prospective Cohort Study," *American Journal of Epidemiology* 177, no. 11 (2013): 1271–8, doi.org/10.1093/aje/kws393.

123 **As a group, Black women:** Latoya Hill, Samantha Artiga, and Usha Ranji, "Racial Disparities in Maternal and Infant Health: Current Status and Efforts to Address Them," KFF, November 1, 2022, kff.org/racial-equity-and -health-policy/issue-brief/racial-disparities-in-maternal-and-infant-health -current-status-and-efforts-to-address-them/.

123 **While socioeconomic factors:** Cristina Novoa and Jamila Taylor, "Exploring African Americans' High Maternal and Infant Death Rates," Center for American Progress, February 1, 2018, americanprogress.org/article /exploring-african-americans-high-maternal-infant-death-rates/.

128 **In July 2021:** Homeland Security Today, "HHS Announces $103 Million from American Rescue Plan to Strengthen Resiliency and Address Burnout in the Health Workforce," US Department of Health & Human Services, August 5, 2021, hstoday.us/subject-matter-areas/mental-health-resilience /hhs-announces-103-million-from-american-rescue-plan-to-strengthen -resiliency-and-address-burnout-in-the-health-workforce/.

CHAPTER 8   A TALE OF TWO EMERGENCY ROOMS

136 **My other shifts:** Brian Fiani et al., "Bellevue Hospital, the Oldest Public Health Center in the United States of America," *World Neurosurgery* 167 (2022): 57–61, doi.org/10.1016/j.wneu.2022.08.088.

137 **In 2010, the year:** Samantha Artiga et al., "Health Coverage by Race and Ethnicity, 2010–2021," KFF, December 20, 2022, kff.org/racial-equity-and -health-policy/issue-brief/health-coverage-by-race-and-ethnicity/.

142 **I believe that:** Elizabeth Whitman, "New York City's Segregated Hospital System," *Modern Healthcare*, February 3, 2017, modernhealthcare.com /article/20170203/NEWS/170209962/new-york-city-s-segregated -hospital-system; Neil Calman et al., "Separate and Unequal: Medical Apartheid in New York City," Institute for Urban Family Health, Bronx Health REACH (2005), nyccoalitiontodismantleracism.files.wordpress.com /2016/03/separate-and-unequal-medical-apartheid-in-new-york-city.pdf.

143 **To this day, only 9 percent:** Barbara Caress, "Hospital Care in Black and White: How Systemic Racism Persists," Center for New York City Affairs at the New School, September 16, 2020, centernyc.org/urban-matters-2/2020/9 /15/hospital-care-in-black-and-white-how-systemic-racism-persists-saved.

143 **Across the nation:** Roosa Sofia Tikkanen et al., "Hospital Payer and Ra-cial/Ethnic Mix at Private Academic Medical Centers in Boston and New York City," *International Journal of Social Determinants of Health and Health Services* 47, no. 3 (2017): 460–76, doi.org/10.1177/0020731416689549.

143 **Uninsured patients are:** Whitman, "New York City's Segregated Hospital System."

143 **What is true:** "2022 Winning Hospitals: Racial Inclusivity," Lown Insti-tute Hospitals Index, accessed December 5, 2022, lownhospitalsindex.org /2022-winning-hospitals-racial-inclusivity/.

143 **A recent study found:** Karen E. Lasser et al., "Changes in Hospitalizations at US Safety-Net Hospitals Following Medicaid Expansion," *JAMA Network Open* 4, no. 6 (2021): e2114343, doi.org/10.1001/jamanetworkopen.2021 .14343.

143 **Even when a top-ranked:** Dan Diamond, "How the Cleveland Clinic Grows Healthier While Its Neighbors Stay Sick," *Politico*, July 17, 2017, politico .com/interactives/2017/obamacare-cleveland-clinic-non-profit-hospital -taxes/.

CHAPTER 9 MOTHERHOOD

151 **Even US Representative:** Laura Olson, "Cori Bush Testified before Con-gress about Black Maternal Deaths, Pregnancy Complications," St. Louis Public Radio, NPR, May 8, 2021, news.stlpublicradio.org/government -politics-issues/2021-05-08/cori-bush-testified-before-congress-about -black-maternal-deaths-pregnancy-complications.

152 **To this day, the United States:** Roosa Tikkanen et al., "Maternal Mortality and Maternity Care in the United States Compared to 10 Other Developed Countries," Commonwealth Fund, November 18, 2020, commonwealthfund .org/publications/issue-briefs/2020/nov/maternal-mortality-maternity -care-us-compared-10-countries.

152 **These numbers are:** "Black Women over Three Times More Likely to Die in Pregnancy, Postpartum Than White Women, New Research Finds," Population Reference Bureau, December 6, 2021, prb.org/resources/black -women-over-three-times-more-likely-to-die-in-pregnancy-postpartum -than-white-women-new-research-finds/.

152 **In NYC, where:** "Pregnancy-Associated Mortality in New York City, 2018," Maternal Mortality Annual Report 2021, New York City Department of Health and Mental Hygiene, January 2022, nyc.gov/assets/doh/downloads /pdf/data/maternal-mortality-annual-report-2021.pdf.

152 **When compared with white:** "Preterm Birth," Centers for Disease Control and Prevention, accessed December 5, 2022, cdc.gov/reproductivehealth /maternalinfanthealth/pretermbirth.htm.

152 **A survey from 2019:** Saraswathi Vedam et al., "The Giving Voice to Mothers Study: Inequity and Mistreatment during Pregnancy and Childbirth in the United States," *Reproductive Health* 16, no. 77 (2019), doi.org/10.1186 /s12978-019-0729-2.

158 **Black women are more likely to be:** "Women's Health Insurance Coverage," KFF, December 21, 2022, kff.org/womens-health-policy/fact-sheet /womens-health-insurance-coverage/.

158 **What's more, Black birthing people:** Katherine M. Jones et al., "Racial and Ethnic Disparities in Breastfeeding," *Breastfeeding Medicine* 10, no. 4 (2015): 186–96, doi.org/10.1089/bfm.2014.0152; Shauna Hemingway et al., "Racial Disparities in Sustaining Breastfeeding in a Baby-Friendly Designated Southeastern United States Hospital: An Opportunity to Investigate Systemic Racism," *Breastfeeding Medicine* 16, no. 2 (2021): 150–5, doi.org /10.1089/bfm.2020.0306; Angela Johnson et al., "Enhancing Breastfeeding Rates among African American Women: A Systematic Review of Current Psychosocial Interventions," *Breastfeeding Medicine* 10, no. 1 (2015): 45–62, doi.org/10.1089/bfm.2014.0023.

160 **Today, doulas are:** Courtney L. Everson, Melissa Cheyney, and Marit L. Bovbjerg, "Outcomes of Care for 1,892 Doula-Supported Adolescent Births in the United States: The DONA International Data Project, 2000 to 2013," *Journal of Perinatal Education* 27, no. 3 (2018): 135–47, doi.org/10.1891 /1058-1243.27.3.135; Katy Backes Kozhimannil et al., "Doula Care, Birth Outcomes, and Costs among Medicaid Beneficiaries," *American Journal of Public Health* 103, no. 4 (2013): 113–21, doi.org/10.2105/AJPH.2012.301201; Meghan A. Bohren et al., "Continuous Support for Women during Childbirth," *Cochrane Database of Systematic Reviews* 2017, no. 7 (2017), doi.org /10.1002/14651858.CD003766.pub6; Ellen D. Hodnett et al., "Continuous Support for Women during Childbirth," *Cochrane Database of Systematic Reviews* 2011, no. 2 (2011), doi.org/10.1002/14651858.CD003766.pub3; Jun Zhang, et al., "Continuous Labor Support from Labor Attendant for Primiparous Women: A Meta-analysis," *Obstetrics & Gynecology* 88, no. 4, part 2 (1996): 739–44, doi.org/10.1016/0029-7844(96)00232-3.

160 **The term is of ancient:** Sam Roberts, "Dana Raphael, Proponent of Breast-Feeding and Use of Doulas, Dies at 90," *New York Times,* February 19, 2016, nytimes.com/2016/02/21/nyregion/dana-raphael-proponent-of-breast-feeding-and-the-use-of-doulas-dies-at-90.html.

161 **In fact, there is a long:** "The Historical Significance of Doulas and Midwives," National Museum of African American History & Culture, accessed December 5, 2022, nmaahc.si.edu/explore/stories/historical-significance-doulas-and-midwives; Keisha La'Nesha Goode, "Birthing, Blackness, and the Body: Black Midwives and Experiential Continuities of Institutional Racism" (PhD diss., City University of New York, 2014).

161 **That all changed:** Judith P. Rooks, *Midwifery and Childbirth in America* (Philadelphia: Temple University Press, 1997).

162 **In 1921, the Sheppard-Towner:** Jillian M. Duquaine-Watson, "Sheppard-Towner Maternity and Infancy Protection Act of 1921," in *The Social History of the American Family: An Encyclopedia,* eds. Marilyn J. Coleman and Lawrence H. Ganong (Thousand Oaks, CA: SAGE Publications, 2014), 1181–3.

162 **In fact, a New York:** Paul Theerman, "Maternal Mortality in New York City: NYAM's Landmark 1933 Study," Center for the History of Medicine and Public Health, New York Academy of Medicine Library, March 7, 2022, nyamcenterforhistory.org/2022/03/07/maternal-mortality-in-new-york-city-nyams-landmark-1933-study/.

162 **In 1900, the United States:** Neelu Shruti, "Black Mothers Matter," *Indypendent,* no. 264, May 25, 2021, https://indypendent.org/2021/05/black-mothers-matter/; Judy Barrett Litoff, "Forgotten Women: American Midwives at the Turn of the Twentieth Century," *Historian* 40, no. 2 (1978): 235–51, jstor.org/stable/24444852.

162 **An abundance of studies:** Andrea Nove et al., "Potential Impact of Midwives in Preventing and Reducing Maternal and Neonatal Mortality and Stillbirths: A Lives Saved Tool Modelling Study," *Lancet Global Health* 9, no. 1 (2021): 24–32, doi.org/10.1016/S2214-109X(20)30397-1; Kiattisak Kongwattanakul et al., "Risk of Severe Adverse Maternal and Neonatal Outcomes in Deliveries with Repeated and Primary Cesarean Deliveries versus Vaginal Deliveries: A Cross-Sectional Study," *Journal of Pregnancy* 2020, no. 9207431 (2020), doi.org/10.1155/2020/9207431; Walid Makin Fahmy, Cibele Aparecida Crispim, and Susan Cliffe, "Association between Maternal Death and Cesarean Section in Latin America: A Systematic Literature Review," *Midwifery* 59 (2018): 88–93, doi.org/10.1016/j.midw.2018.01.009; Rayhan Sk, "Does Delivery in Private Hospitals Contribute Largely to Caesarean Section Births? A Path Analysis Using Generalised Structural Equation Modelling," *PLoS One* 15, no. 10 (2020): e0239649, doi.org/10.1371/journal.pone.0239649; J. J. Zwart et al., "Severe Maternal Morbidity during Pregnancy, Delivery and Puerperium in the Netherlands: A Nationwide Population-Based Study of 371,000 Pregnancies," *BJOG* 115, no. 7 (2008): 842–50, doi.org/10.1111/j.1471-0528.2008.01713.x; Olivia

Dockery, "Honoring Black Birth Workers of the Past," HealthConnect One, February 6, 2020, healthconnectone.org/honoring-black-birth-workers-of -the-past/; Vivienne Souter et al., "Comparison of Midwifery and Obstetric Care in Low-Risk Hospital Births," *Obstetrics & Gynecology* 134, no. 5 (2019): 1056–65, doi.org/10.1097/AOG.0000000000003521.

162 **Midwifery has been:** Margaret Hanahoe, "Midwifery-Led Care Can Lower Caesarean Section Rates According to the Robson Ten Group Classification System," *European Journal of Midwifery* 4, no. 7 (2020), doi.org /10.18332/ejm/119164.

162 **In 2018, however:** Michaeleen Doucleff, "Rate of C-Sections Is Rising at an 'Alarming' Rate, Report Says," *Goats and Soda*, NPR, October 12, 2018, npr .org/sections/goatsandsoda/2018/10/12/656198429/rate-of-c-sections-is -rising-at-an-alarming-rate.

163 **Meanwhile, a full:** National Academies of Sciences, Engineering, and Medicine, *Birth Settings in America: Outcomes, Quality, Access, and Choice* (Washington, DC: National Academies Press, 2020), doi.org/10.17226 /25636; Joyce A. Martin et al., "Births: Final Data for 2006," *National Vital Statistics Reports* 57, no. 7 (2009), cdc.gov/nchs/data/nvsr/nvsr57/nvsr57 _07.pdf.

163 **For example, 69 percent:** Eugene R. Declercq et al., *Listening to Mothers III: Pregnancy and Birth,* Childbirth Connection (2013), nationalpartnership .org/our-work/resources/health-care/maternity/listening-to-mothers -iii-pregnancy-and-birth-2013.pdf.

163 **I felt incredibly fortunate:** Paula M. Lantz et al., "Doulas as Childbirth Paraprofessionals: Results from a National Survey," *Women's Health Issues* 15, no. 3 (2005): 109–16, doi.org/10.1016/j.whi.2005.01.002.

163 **For many doulas of color:** Rachel R. Hardeman and Katy B. Kozhimannil, "Motivations for Entering the Doula Profession: Perspectives from Women of Color," *Journal of Midwifery & Women's Health* 61, no. 6 (2016): 773–80, doi.org/10.1111/jmwh.12497.

165 **Every now and again:** Minyvonne Burke, "Death of Black Mother after Birth of First Child Highlights Racial Disparities in Maternal Mortality," NBC News, November 6, 2020, nbcnews.com/news/us-news/death-black -mother-after-birth-first-child-highlights-racial-disparities-n1246841.

165 **Or Sha-Asia Washington:** Alyssa Newcomb, "Pregnant 26-Year-Old's Death Sheds Light on Health Care System That Fails Black Mothers," *Today,* July 15, 2020, today.com/health/death-sha-asia-washington-sheds-light-racial -disparities-black-mothers-t186898.

165 **Work is being:** Cheyanne M. Daniels, "Lawmakers Push to End Maternal Health Crisis," *The Hill,* November 4, 2022, thehill.com/policy/3719457 -lawmakers-push-to-end-maternal-health-crisis/; "About the Black Maternal Health Momnibus Act of 2021," United States House of Representative Black Maternal Health Caucus, accessed December 5, 2022, blackmaternalhealthcaucus-underwood.house.gov/Momnibus.

166 **acknowledges that doulas:** "About the Black Maternal Health Momnibus Act of 2021."

166 **A 2019 study of a Black-owned:** Rachel R. Hardeman et al., "Roots Community Birth Center: A Culturally-Centered Care Model for Improving Value and Equity in Childbirth," *Healthcare* 8, no. 1 (2020), doi.org/10.1016/j.hjdsi.2019.100367.

CHAPTER 10   DIVERSITY AND EXCLUSION

171 **A recent study revealed:** "Diversity in Medicine: Facts and Figures 2019," Association of American Medical Colleges, accessed December 5, 2022, aamc.org/data-reports/workforce/report/diversity-medicine-facts-and-figures-2019.

CHAPTER 11   TRUTH TO POWER

190 **Concurrently, national studies:** National Academies of Sciences, Engineering, and Medicine, *Sexual Harassment of Women: Climate, Culture, and Consequences in Academic Sciences, Engineering, and Medicine* (Washington, DC: National Academies Press, 2018), ncbi.nlm.nih.gov/books/NBK519462/.

203 **University of Georgia professor:** Kevin Donahue et al., "The Infuriating Journey from Pet to Threat: How Bias Undermines Black Women at Work," *Forbes EQ*, June 29, 2021, forbes.com/sites/forbeseq/2021/06/29/the-infuriating-journey-from-pet-to-threat-how-bias-undermines-black-women-at-work/?sh=45fa8e556490.

CHAPTER 12   ALL THE PATIENTS LOOK LIKE US

217 **My observation was:** Kevin Quealy, "The Richest Neighborhoods Emptied Out Most as Coronavirus Hit New York City," *New York Times*, May 15, 2020, nytimes.com/interactive/2020/05/15/upshot/who-left-new-york-coronavirus.html.

224 **The pandemic was making:** Richard A. Oppel Jr. et al., "The Fullest Look Yet at the Racial Inequity of Coronavirus," *New York Times*, July 5, 2020, nytimes.com/interactive/2020/07/05/us/coronavirus-latinos-african-americans-cdc-data.html; John Eligon et al., "Black Americans Face Alarming Rates of Coronavirus Infection in Some States," *New York Times*, published April 7, 2020, updated April 14, 2020, nytimes.com/2020/04/07/us/coronavirus-race.html; Brian M. Rosenthal et al., "Why Surviving the Virus Might Come Down to Which Hospital Admits You," *New York Times*, published July 1, 2020, updated September 22, 2021, nytimes.com/2020/07/01/nyregion/Coronavirus-hospitals.html; Michael Schwirtz, "One Rich N.Y. Hospital Got Warren Buffett's Help. This One Got Duct Tape," *New York Times*, published April 26, 2020, updated May 20, 2020,

nytimes.com/2020/04/26/nyregion/coronavirus-new-york-university
-hospital.html.

225 **In the first half of 2020:** Oni Blackstock and Uché Blackstock, "Black
Americans Should Face Lower Age Cutoffs to Qualify for a Vaccine," *Washington Post*, February 19, 2021, washingtonpost.com/opinions/black-americans
-should-face-lower-age-cutoffs-to-qualify-for-a-vaccine/2021/02/19
/3029d5de-72ec-11eb-b8a9-b9467510f0fe_story.html.

CHAPTER 13   WHERE I'M SUPPOSED TO BE

230 **Even the chronic stress:** Arline T. Geronimus et al., "'Weathering' and Age
Patterns of Allostatic Load Scores among Blacks and Whites in the United
States," *American Journal of Public Health* 96, no. 5 (2006): 826–33, doi
.org/10.2105/AJPH.2004.060749.

232 **In the US, around:** Ian Thomsen, "1,000 People in the U.S. Die Every Year
in Police Shootings. Who Are They?" *Northeastern Global News*, April 16,
2020, news.northeastern.edu/2020/04/16/000-people-in-the-us-are-killed
-every-year-in-police-shootings-how-many-are-preventable/.

232 **Black Americans are three:** "Black People More Than Three Times As Likely
As White People to Be Killed during a Police Encounter," Harvard T. H.
Chan School of Public Health, accessed December 5, 2022, hsph.harvard
.edu/news/hsph-in-the-news/blacks-whites-police-deaths-disparity/.

232 **Statistics from a 2018:** Frank Edwards, Hedwig Lee, and Michael Esposito, "Risk of Being Killed by Police Use of Force in the United States by
Age, Race-Ethnicity, and Sex," *Proceedings of the National Academy of Sciences* 116, no. 34 (2019): 16793–8, doi.org/10.1073/pnas.1821204116.

232 **Yet recent research:** Sirry Alang, Donna D. McAlpine, and Rachel Hardeman, "Police Brutality and Mistrust in Medical Institutions," *Journal of
Racial and Ethnic Health Disparities* 7, no. 4 (2020): 760–8, doi.org/10.1007
/s40615-020-00706-w.

232 **One study suggests:** Rachel R. Hardeman et al., "Association of Residence
in High-Police Contact Neighborhoods with Preterm Birth among Black
and White Individuals in Minneapolis," *JAMA Network Open* 4, no. 12 (2021):
e2130290, doi.org/10.1001/jamanetworkopen.2021.30290.

236 **The US is the wealthiest:** Eric C. Schneider et al., *Mirror, Mirror 2021: Reflecting Poorly: Health Care in the U.S. Compared to Other High-Income
Countries* (New York: Commonwealth Fund, 2021), commonwealthfund
.org/sites/default/files/2021-08/Schneider_Mirror_Mirror_2021.pdf.

236 **In December 2020:** John Eligon, "Black Doctor Dies of Covid-19 after
Complaining of Racist Treatment," *New York Times*, published December
23, 2020, updated December 25, 2020, nytimes.com/2020/12/23/us/susan
-moore-black-doctor-indiana.html.

237 **Not only have white:** Michael W. Sjoding et al., "Racial Bias in Pulse Oxim-

etry Measurement," Letter to the Editor, *New England Journal of Medicine* 383 (2020): 2477–8, doi.org/10.1056/NEJMc2029240.

CHAPTER 14 A BETTER WAY

240 **Access was an issue:** Wilson Majee et al., "The Past Is So Present: Understanding COVID-19 Vaccine Hesitancy among African American Adults Using Qualitative Data," *Journal of Racial and Ethnic Health Disparities* 10 (2023): 462–74, doi.org/10.1007/s40615-022-01236-3.

240 **Due to systemic:** Majee et al., "The Past Is So Present."

242 **In 2018, about 55 percent:** Edward R. Berchick, Jessica C. Barnett, and Rachel D. Upton, "Health Insurance Coverage in the United States: 2018," United States Census Bureau, Report Number P60-267 (RV), November 8, 2019, census.gov/library/publications/2019/demo/p60-267.html.

242 **The very first vaccine:** Gillian Brockell, "The African Roots of Inoculation in America: Saving Lives for Three Centuries," *Washington Post*, December 15, 2020, washingtonpost.com/history/2020/12/15/enslaved-african-smallpox-vaccine-coronavirus/.

242 **Onesimus explained the principle:** Erin Blakemore, "How an Enslaved African Man in Boston Helped Save Generations from Smallpox," History, published February 1, 2019, updated April 8, 2021, history.com/news/smallpox-vaccine-onesimus-slave-cotton-mather.

243 **A Confederate doctor:** Jim Downs, "Never Forget That Early Vaccines Came from Testing on Enslaved People," *STAT*, June 19, 2022, statnews.com/2022/06/19/never-forget-that-early-vaccines-came-from-testing-on-enslaved-people/.

244 **But the Biden-Harris:** Oni Blackstock and Uché Blackstock, "Black Americans Should Face Lower Age Cutoffs to Qualify for a Vaccine," *Washington Post*, February 19, 2021, washingtonpost.com/opinions/black-americans-should-face-lower-age-cutoffs-to-qualify-for-a-vaccine/2021/02/19/3029d5de-72ec-11eb-b8a9-b9467510f0fe_story.html.

247 **By then, Congress:** Sharon Parrott et al., "CARES Act Includes Essential Measures to Respond to Public Health, Economic Crises, but More Will Be Needed," Center on Budget and Policy Priorities, March 27, 2020, cbpp.org/research/economy/cares-act-includes-essential-measures-to-respond-to-public-health-economic-crises.

247 **Later, we learned:** Rachel Garfield, Kendal Orgera, and Anthony Damico, "The Coverage Gap: Uninsured Poor Adults in States That Do Not Expand Medicaid," KFF, January 21, 2021, kff.org/medicaid/issue-brief/the-coverage-gap-uninsured-poor-adults-in-states-that-do-not-expand-medicaid/.

248 **Experts in infectious:** Stan Dorn and Rebecca Gordon, "The Catastrophic Cost of Uninsurance: COVID-19 Cases and Deaths Closely Tied to America's Health Coverage Gaps," Families USA, March 4, 2021, familiesusa

.org/resources/the-catastrophic-cost-of-uninsurance-covid-19-cases
-and-deaths-closely-tied-to-americas-health-coverage-gaps/.

248 **According to CDC:** Robin A. Cohen at al., "Health Insurance Coverage: Early Release of Estimates from the National Health Interview Survey, January–June 2021," National Center for Health Statistics, November 2021, cdc.gov/nchs/data/nhis/earlyrelease/insur202111.pdf.

248 **The closest we:** Jeneen Interlandi, "Why Doesn't the United States Have Universal Health Care? The Answer Has Everything to Do with Race," *New York Times Magazine*, August 14, 2019, https://nyti.ms/2HMLO9P; "A Brief History: Universal Health Care Efforts in the US," Physicians for a National Health Program, accessed December 5, 2022, pnhp.org/a-brief-history -universal-health-care-efforts-in-the-us/; Dr. Howard Markel, "69 Years Ago, a President Pitches His Idea for National Health Care," PBS, November 19, 2014, pbs.org/newshour/health/november-19-1945-harry-truman -calls-national-health-insurance-program.

250 **Black organizations have:** Vann R. Newkirk II, "The Fight for Health Care Has Always Been about Civil Rights," *Atlantic*, June 27, 2017, theatlantic .com/politics/archive/2017/06/the-fight-for-health-care-is-really-all -about-civil-rights/531855/.

251 **By 2018, the uninsured:** Berchick, Barnett, and Upton, "Health Insurance Coverage in the United States: 2018."

251 **A 2022 study:** Rachel Nuwer, "Universal Health Care Could Have Saved More Than 330,000 U.S. Lives during COVID," *Scientific American*, June 13, 2022, scientificamerican.com/article/universal-health-care-could-have -saved-more-than-330-000-u-s-lives-during-covid/.

252 **As I write this:** Selena Simmons-Duffin, "Free COVID Tests and Treatments No Longer Free for Uninsured, As Funding Runs Out," *Shots*, NPR, March 29, 2022, npr.org/sections/health-shots/2022/03/29/1089355997 /free-covid-tests-and-treatments-no-longer-free-for-uninsured-as-funding -runs-out.

CHAPTER 15   THE WAY FORWARD: ACTIONS SPEAK LOUDER THAN WORDS

253 **In March 1955:** Vann R. Newkirk II, "The Fight for Health Care Has Always Been about Civil Rights," *Atlantic*, June 27, 2017, theatlantic.com /politics/archive/2017/06/the-fight-for-health-care-is-really-all-about -civil-rights/531855/.

EPILOGUE

265 **In her essay:** Dale G. Blackstock, "A Black Woman in Medicine," in *Women in Medical Education: An Anthology of Experience*, ed. Delese Wear (Albany: State University of New York Press, 1996), 75–80.

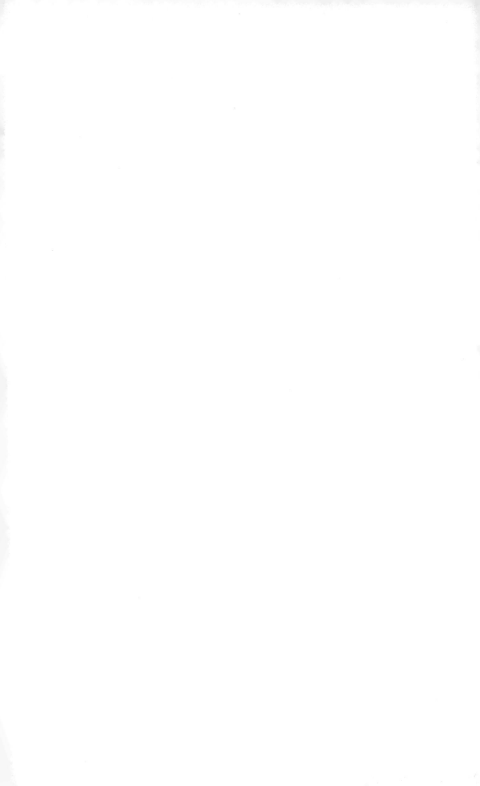